..:::. **INNER BEAUTY** .:::..

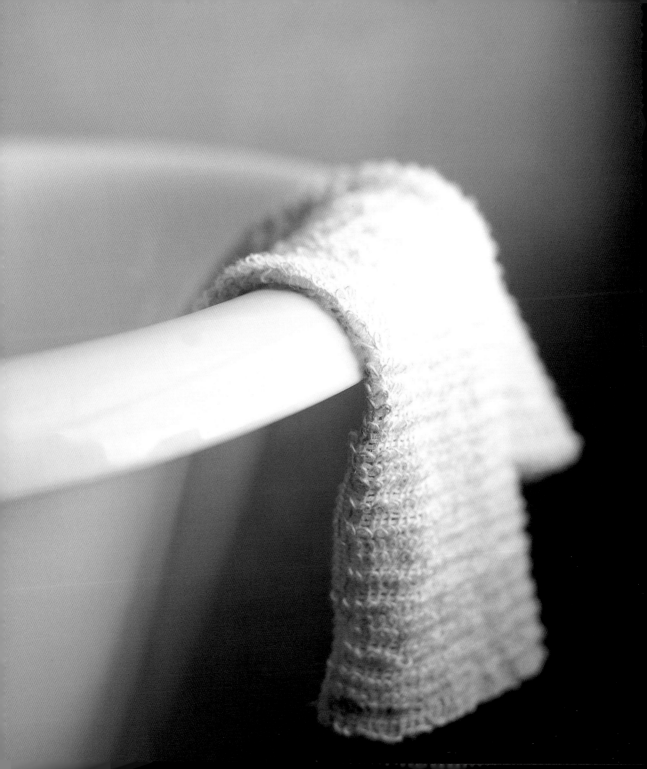

INNER BEAUTY

DISCOVER NATURAL BEAUTY AND WELL-BEING

with the

TRADITIONS OF AYURVEDA

By Reenita Malhotra Hora

Photographs by France Ruffenach

Foreword by William B. Stewart, M.D.

CHRONICLE BOOKS

SAN FRANCISCO

Text copyright © 2005 by Reenita Malhotra Hora.
Photographs copyright © 2005 by France Ruffenach.
Illustration copyright © 2003 by Nicole Kaufman.

Library of Congress Cataloging-in-Publication
Data available.

ISBN 0-8118-4276-2

Manufactured in China.

Styling by Sara Slavin
Design by Sara Schneider

Distributed in Canada by Raincoast Books
9050 Shaughnessy Street
Vancouver, British Columbia V6P 6E5

10 9 8 7 6 5 4 3 2 1

Chronicle Books LLC
85 Second Street
San Francisco, California 94105

www.chroniclebooks.com

Photographer Acknowledgment

*The photographer wishes to thank Reenita Malhotra
Hora for inspirational content; editor Lisa Campbell
for her positive support; Barbara Vick and Carey
Nowell for generously allowing access into their gor-
geous homes; Shawna Moriarty for a graceful lotus
pose; Cedric Glasier for his unmatched support and
knowledge; Sara Slavin for her creativity, spirit, and
perfect sense of style; and Sara Schneider for her constant belief in a shared vision, and commitment to
beautiful design.*

For Neeraj Hora, my best friend and soul mate.

..:.:. ॐ .:.:..

Yaa Devi Sarvabhuteshu Vidyaroopena Sanstitha I
Namastasyai Namstasyai Namastasyai Namo Namah II

My respects to the Goddess who exists in life as Knowledge.

The Markandeya Purana

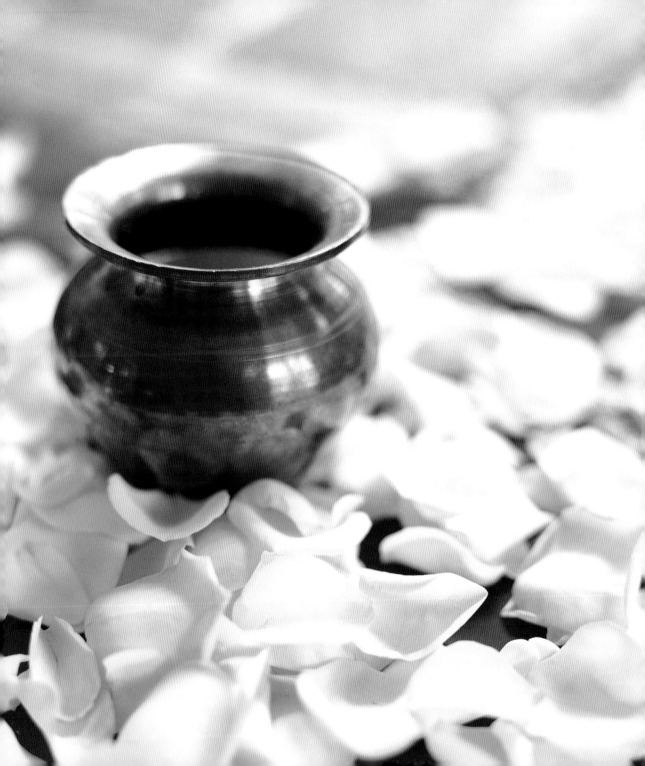

CONTENTS

FOREWORD

Ayurveda is five-thousand-year-old medicine that has much to offer any-one in search of a healthy lifestyle today. The Sanskrit word *Ayurveda* has two roots: *ayur*, meaning life, and *veda*, meaning knowledge. The system-atic collection of health and healing knowledge encompassing all aspects of life and daily living has led the practice of Ayurveda to be called the "science of life." A comprehensive approach, Ayurveda includes concepts of creation and energy, precepts of the moral and ethical life, and recom-mended practices relating to nutrition, physical activity, rest, relaxation, and spiritual practice. It is truly a timeless wisdom practice based on centuries of careful observation and interpretation.

In *Inner Beauty*, Reenita Malhotra Hora gives us a guide to the practice of Ayurveda that yokes ancient wisdom—both knowledge and practices—with contemporary reality. She understands the challenges of modern life and provides facts and routines that are understandable, acces-sible, and doable. She teaches that true well-being and beauty originate within—they cannot be achieved through anything that covers or masks who we truly are. When we feel good, we look good. Feeling good requires a commitment to what we take in (in the form of food and drink, sounds, sights), what we feel (in the form of emotions and sensations), and how we relate to everything around us. Ayurveda is about balance, relatedness, lifelong learning, and daily practice.

Inner Beauty, with its time-tested approaches, practical recom-mendations, and straightforward language, is an invaluable book for all those open to taking responsibility for their own well-being.

WILLIAM B. STEWART, M.D.

MEDICAL DIRECTOR, INSTITUTE FOR HEALTH AND HEALING
CALIFORNIA PACIFIC MEDICAL CENTER
SAN FRANCISCO, CALIFORNIA

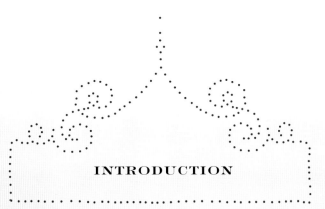

INTRODUCTION

I grew up in Bombay—India's most dynamic city, but still a place steeped in ancient traditions of the oldest living culture known. This contrast was also borne out in my own family, who expected that I would be educated and have a career, but also made sure I was immersed in the culture of Ayurveda, the ancient teachings of health and well-being. I surprised my family by being even more independent than they had taught me to be when I insisted on attending college in the United States. I was set on becoming a marketing professional of some sort. I saw myself as a completely modern woman.

Ayurveda was the furthest thing from my mind when I embarked on this educational adventure. After all, it was just routine to me to practice yoga, to eat triphala with honey at breakfast, or to oil my hair before showering. But something happened when I went to college. In an atmosphere of intense competition and high expectations, I watched many of my friends survive on a never-ending cycle of caffeine and Tylenol. Rather than listening to the demands of their own bodies, as I had been taught to do, they were trying to override their needs for sleep and for good nutrition by using synthetic solutions. And it wasn't working—they told me over and over that they felt tired, stressed out, depleted. It was then that I began to realize how important Ayurveda is for health, for beauty, and for feeling your best, and that I had lived all my life taking the ancient wisdom for granted. So I surprised my family again by deciding to pursue a career in Ayurveda. After I finished college, I decided to study Ayurvedic medicine. I knew I would become a health educator and consultant, and above all, an ambassador for this wonderful, ancient life science that was so much a part of me.

I often ask myself, How did I get to this point? How did I come to this crossroads of so-called modern life and the ancient traditions of Ayurveda? The answer is my family. My late grandfather, Gopal Krishan Vij, made an indelible imprint on my life and values. He was a man who lived simply and sought to achieve his full potential in whatever task he took on, from being a civil engineer to being a father. He encouraged the women of his family to be strong, be smart, and achieve whatever they set out to do. Along with my grandmother, he taught us all the subtle principles of Ayurveda, so that our minds and bodies would always be healthy. My grandfather also discouraged us from vanity and self-indulgence, from devoting our energies to jewelry, makeup, and fashion—he knew there was so much more to life than that.

Under my grandfather's influence, the women of my family defined beauty not as something exterior, like a beautiful dress or sparkling jewels, but rather radiance that comes from health, confidence, and self-esteem. My grandfather would often describe to me his mother, my great-grandmother, who woke early every morning to care for her family and dressed simply in a white sari, her face clean; she was the embodiment of this ideal. Learning from her example, that kind of beauty became my ideal, too. In writing Inner Beauty, my goal was to teach others the principles of Ayurveda so they can cultivate the same radiance, beauty, and well-being that the women of my family demonstrated to me.

The following pages are designed to enable you to achieve inner beauty through a balanced, healthy, Ayurvedic lifestyle. This is a book for anyone who wants to end the cycle of stress and exhaustion and the toll they take on our health and appearance by making simple, sensible lifestyle changes. *Inner Beauty* is an introduction to the principles of Ayurveda, and details how to put them to work. In the first chapter, you'll learn about the philosophy of Ayurveda and how it has evolved from an ancient medicine into a staple of the contemporary Indian household. You'll learn about *ojas*—the life force or vitality that is the source of inner beauty—and the science behind Ayurveda. Chapter Two introduces the *doshas*—the three mind-body energies that are a part of each of us. You'll also learn how to determine which *dosha* is dominant in you, the key to selecting the Ayurvedic treatments, remedies, and regimes—from facial cleansers to yoga routines—that will help you feel balanced and healthy. Chapter Three offers recipes for traditional homemade cleansers and moisturizers for the hair, skin, and body that are customized for your *dosha*, like a soothing Milk and Rice Water Bath (page 60) or an exfoliating cleanser made from herbs you probably already have in your kitchen (page 53). Chapter Four teaches a balanced approach to fitness, focusing on yoga, which shares its origins with Ayurveda. You'll learn how to choose a style of yoga practice that's right for you and the routines that are best for your body type. In Chapter Five, you'll learn the principles of Ayurvedic nutrition and how to make smart choices. Chapter Six describes seasonal practices for well-being, such as an at-home "detox retreat" that will help you recharge your batteries. The last chapter is a guide to professional spa treatments that will enhance your practice of Ayurveda.

Inner Beauty is not only an introduction to Ayurveda, but also potential tool for changing your life for the better by restoring a sense of balance and sanity that is so often missing from our busy lives. The treatments and routines in this book are meant to help you be your best, feel your best, and look your best—in short, to let the inner beauty that is already inside you shine out for all the world to see.

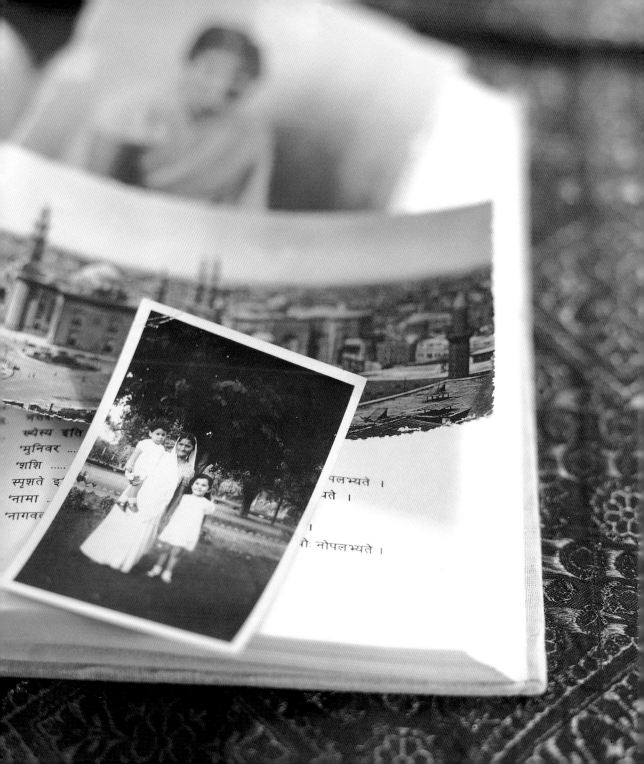

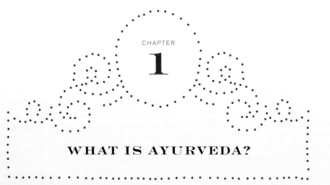

WHAT IS AYURVEDA?

Ayurveda is a five-thousand-year-old healing system from India and the oldest medical science in existence. Sanskrit for "the Science of Life," it is a set of self-care guidelines that will help any person stay healthy and feel good by understanding the needs of his or her own mind and body. Ayurveda is intended to help each person be her best self—healthy, happy, and radiant with beauty. Ayurvedic beauty treatments include skin care, diet, massage, and exercise routines that are customized for every person to reflect their unique needs.

Ayurveda recognizes that we are all different—that each of us has a unique mind and body. After all, we look and behave differently from one another, and we all have different reactions to everyday situations. Everything from the foods we eat to the emotions we experience affect us each in our own way. We all have our own personal definition of what it means to be happy, healthy, and in balance—that is, feeling full of energy and life. And because we are each unique, we will all require different treatments and remedies to help us be our best. Ayurveda as a system includes tools to help figure out what these customized treatments should be.

Ayurveda acknowledges that the mind and body are not two separate entities but are closely intertwined. We've all seen how our thinking affects our body (say, when we're worried or upset and then our skin breaks out) and how our body affects our mind (like the way our self-esteem plummets when we don't get regular exercise). Ayurveda has two special terms to convey this idea. The physical or tangible body, *Sthoola Sharira*, is our skin, bones, muscles—everything you would find in a Western anatomy textbook. The energetic body, *Sukshna Sharira*, is that with which we feel, sense, spiritualize, emote, and think. So happiness and joy, emotional pain, psyche, perceptions, hunches, and intuition are all considered to form part of our energetic anatomy. Ayurveda works on healing both the energetic and the physical bodies, because one can never reach its full potential if the other is not strong.

Ayurveda teaches us how to stay healthy and balanced. Ayurvedic treatments—from digestive herbal teas to oil massages and facials—are intended to be gentle habits that can last a lifetime, not extreme regimes or quick fixes. Ayurveda is unlike many other health systems, which oversimplify the variety of factors that affect our health and how we feel and only address the symptoms, not the causes, of imbalance. Because many of us experience so much stress these days, and because "feeling stressed" is really just another way of saying our life is out of balance, Ayurveda is more useful and important than ever before. It's the perfect antidote to stress because it addresses the whole person and how she is affected by her lifestyle.

.:.:.:.:. THE ORIGINS OF AYURVEDA .:.:.:.:.

Though its origins are lost to historians, Ayurveda is believed to have come from the Vedic gods over five thousand years ago, when a group of scholars and mystics met in the Himalayas to try to discover the secrets of longevity and the cures for illnesses of every kind. Through meditation and spiritual communion with the gods, the scholars and mystics arrived upon guidance for everything from everyday well-being to internal medicine and surgery. Ayurveda was an oral tradition in India for hundreds of years, until it was collected into three main texts: the *Charak Samhita*, the *Sushrut Samhita*, and the *Ashtanga Hridayam*. (The exact dates of authorship are not known, but the *Charak Samhita* and the *Sushrut Samhita* are thought to have been written in the first few centuries BCE, with the *Ashtangu Hridayam* coming later, about 400 CE.) The books are written in Sanskrit verse (Sanskrit is the ancient language of India, just as Latin is to the Western world). This vivid poetry articulates Ayurvedic philosophies and concepts. For this reason, it's hard to define whether Ayurveda is an art or a science. It might well in fact be both, as the Sanskrit verses reflect both on the theoretical aspects of Ayurveda—the art side—and the practical knowledge involved in incorporating it into human lives.

Traditionally, most Indian villages had their own Ayurvedic doctor, who would advise the community about self-care practices and gather medicinal plants from the surrounding forests. This doctor would explain the meanings of the Ayurvedic sutras, or teachings, to student apprentices, who then prepared and dispensed medicines according to his instruction. In the years when India was a colony of the British Empire, the ruling powers tried to stop the practice of Ayurveda (amongst other traditional medicines) and it temporarily lost the cultural influence it once held. But after India became an independent nation in 1947, Ayurveda began to undergo a renaissance, and has since become popular all over the world.

Today, Ayurveda is a part of everyday life in many Indian households. For example, families drink water or water-based drinks that have been stored in a copper vessel, because Ayurveda recognizes that copper detoxifies the body and boosts the immune system. The sacred basil plant tulsi, offered in prayer to the Indian god Lord Vishnu, is typically placed in the central area of Indian homes to clarify the mind of impure thoughts, and to rid the environment of microbes. Finally, herbal kitchen remedies form a natural part of every Indian housewife's repertoire: common culinary items like turmeric, ginger, and dairy cream are used for beauty treatments and to heal minor ailments.

.:.:.:.:. **HOW AYURVEDA WORKS** .:.:.:.:.

Ayurveda teaches that health and beauty are the results of a powerful energy within us. The more of that energy we have in us, the better we look and feel. Maximizing this energy is the essential goal of Ayurveda. This energy is called *ojas* (pronounced oh-*jus*), which means "that which invigorates." It is the life force, the energy that flows through every person and living thing. Like chi in Chinese philosophy, *ojas* is the force that makes us feel happy and alive. Responsible for wellness, harmony, and spiritual growth, it makes our eyes shine and puts a spring in our step. High levels of *ojas* bring bliss and happiness, which those around us see as radiance, poise, a glowing complexion, and a sharp intellect—in short, inner beauty.

Ojas connects people and living things, and is present in every aspect of life, from our emotional well-being to the foods we eat. For example, soil with strong *ojas* is rich in nutrients. It has the capacity to nurture a healthy apple tree that will root itself deep in the ground and grow to substantial heights. Filled with a high level of *ojas*, this tree bears lush and nutritious fruit. The woman who eats the fruit absorbs not only vitamins, but *ojas*, which provides strength and longevity to her mind and body. When her own *ojas* potential is maximized, this woman is energized, inspiring everyone around her. The wheel turns full circle when the apple core goes into the compost heap and is recycled back into the environment, feeding the soil that gave life to the original tree.

When *ojas* is low we are like dried leaves—tired, worn out, and brittle. We experience a breakdown in the normal functions of our mind-body system and become susceptible to illness, both emotionally and physically. The best way to keep our *ojas* up is to live a balanced lifestyle that is pure and close to nature. An overactive lifestyle (known as *rajas*) or a dull, inert lifestyle (known as *tamas*) both cause stress and deplete

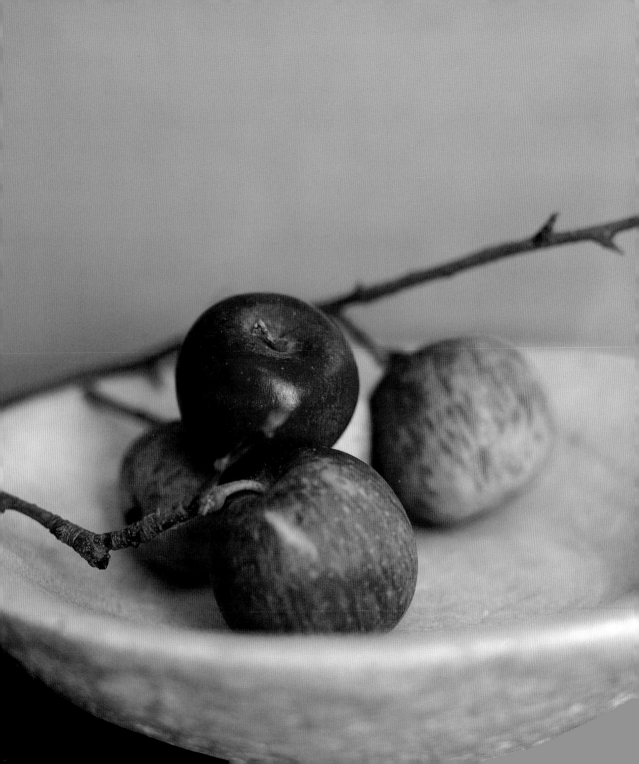

ojas. We must strive for a state of purity and balance, a third way of life called *sattwa.* Ayurvedic routines for personal care, both on a daily basis (called *dinacharya*) and seasonally (called *ritucharya*), help us stay in balance. Inner beauty will unfold naturally if you protect the mind and body against unhealthy influences and live in harmony with the natural laws of the universe.

.:.:.:.:. **THE BUILDING BLOCKS OF BALANCE** .:.:.:.:.

We know that living in balance is the key to achieving and maintaining high *ojas,* the ultimate destination of our Ayurvedic journey. But what does it mean to live in balance? Ayurveda teaches that each of us is a unique individual, in the way we think, move, act, how we react to stress, in the foods we like to eat, and in the activities we enjoy. So balance will mean something different for each person. Ayurveda will help you determine the makeup of your mind and body—your natural tendencies and preferences. With this knowledge, it's a simple step to learn what to do (and what not to do) to even out those characteristics and achieve balance.

Ayurveda tells us that each person, like the world itself, is composed of five elements: space, air, fire, water, and earth. The qualities of these elements are apparent in our physical bodies and our energetic bodies. For example, the light and mobile quality of air gives us the ability both to move our bodies and to be flexible in our thinking. The smooth and liquid quality of water gives sheen to our hair and makes for a nurturing disposition. But these five elements do not exist separately within us. Instead, they unite to form three distinct energetic forces, called *doshas.* Each *dosha* is a combination of two of these five elements, and all are present to some degree in each person.

Air, which provides movement, and space, which provides vastness, unite to form the *vata dosha,* which has an overall light, cold, dry, and dispersing quality. *Vata* initiates movement in the mind—thoughts, ideas, and creativity—and also physical movement in the body, impulses in our nervous system, our blood and lymphatic circulation, walking, and even gesturing with our hands.

Fire, which provides heat, and water, which provides fluidity, unite to form the *pitta dosha*, which has an overall heating, oily, sharp, and penetrating quality. *Pitta* controls transformations in the mind such as intelligence, reasoning, passion, and the operation of the senses, as well as physical transformations such as metabolism, hormonal activity, enzymatic behavior, and body temperature.

Water together with earth, which provides solidity, unite to form the *kapha dosha*, which has an overall heavy, cold, oily, and cohesive property. *Kapha* provides nurturing and lubrication to the mind, and helps preserve our memory. It also binds and lubricates our physical tissues with mucus, body fluids, and plasma, making the body stable and firm.

The individual proportions of the three *doshas* in each person is called *prakruti*, or mind-body constitution. Understanding your *prakruti* is like knowing how to read the blueprint for your own house. Although a complete understanding of your *prakruti* is gained through meeting with an experienced Ayurvedic professional, in the next chapter, you will learn more about *prakruti*, the three *doshas*, and how to get a sense of what your own dominant *dosha* might be, which is the first step towards Ayurvedic healing.

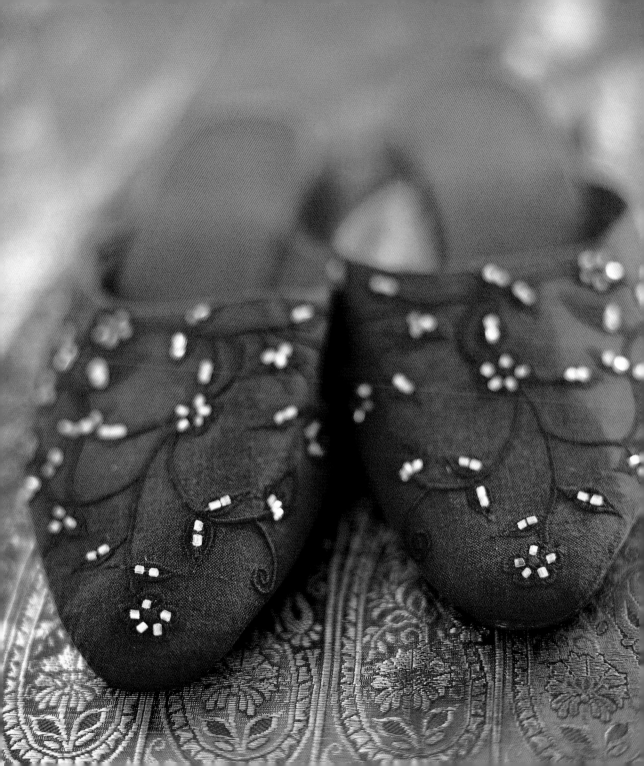

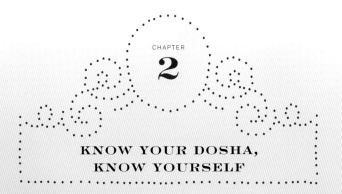

CHAPTER

2

KNOW YOUR DOSHA,
KNOW YOURSELF

The Ayurvedic concept of *prakruti*, which translates literally from Sanskrit as "nature," refers to our natural mind-body constitution—the unique characteristics that each of us is born with, perceptible through emotions, behavior, body type, metabolism, and health tendencies. The overall nature of a person's constitution is largely determined by which of the *doshas* (*vata*, *pitta*, or *kapha*) is predominant. All three *doshas* exist in varying levels in each of us. Imagine a pie chart with three sections—these proportions are different for each person, but always add up to 100 percent.

Most of us comprise more of one *dosha* than the other two, and our emotional capacities, physical characteristics, and behavior will mostly reflect the qualities of the dominant *dosha*. Some of us exhibit more than one of the *dosha* characteristics, in that two of the three *doshas* exist more or less equally in a higher proportion relative to the third. These are "mixed *dosha*" types. It is quite common, for example, to be a *vata-pitta* type, exhibiting the physical and emotional characteristics of both *doshas*. In other cases, one *dosha* might dominate physical traits and another *dosha* show itself in emotional traits, or both characteristics could be a mix of both *doshas*. Very few people will actually have equal proportions of all three *doshas*, making them "tri-*dosha*" types. For the purposes of this book you'll identify the one predominant *dosha* that characterizes your mind and body and what to do to keep that *dosha* in balance.

To increase *ojas*, our core energy, we need to constantly balance our *prakruti*, our essential nature. So understanding *prakruti* and the elements that compose it becomes the natural first step in our journey to cultivate inner beauty. While everybody is born with a basic *prakruti* that is unique and will stay constant through life, the day-to-day interplay of *dosha* tendencies are likely to vary based upon influences from food, lifestyle, environment, and seasons. We can examine our lifestyles to see whether we are "living right" and maintaining balance, or whether our lifestyle is driving any *doshas* into excess. Once this happens, we can begin to use the diet, skin-care regimen, and fitness programs or yoga techniques that work best to keep us in balance.

As *prakruti* varies from individual to individual, so does the definition of balance. As stated earlier, according to Ayurveda, balance does not mean "all things being equal," or all of us having equal amounts of each *dosha* within us. Instead, it is a state of equilibrium wherein our current *dosha* levels match the specific proportions of our natural mind-body makeup. When in equilibrium, the *doshas* help us be our best selves. But when they go out of balance, they create problems such as sluggishness, dehydration, inflammation, and other sensitivities. If you consider that *dosha* literally translates from Sanskrit as "that which easily goes off balance," it becomes clear that staying in balance is a challenge for us all.

When first introduced to the concept, many ask the question, Which of the *doshas* is the best? In fact, they are all the best when they are balanced, and they are all the worst when they are imbalanced. No matter what our *dosha*, the goal is to bring it into balance and live closest to *prakruti*, our natural state of inner beauty.

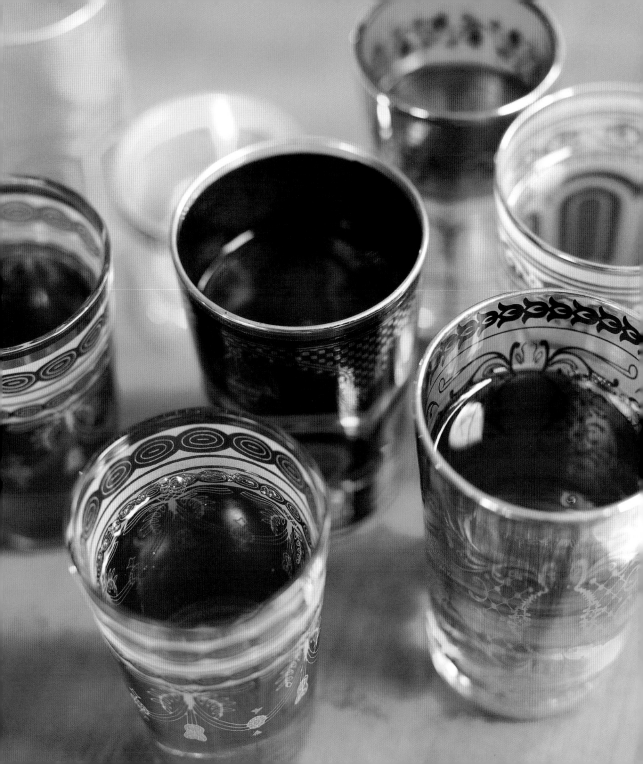

VATA

The characteristics of *vata* (air and space) can be likened to those of a desert or outer space—a vast amount of space with air moving though it. Unobstructed, the air can change its course with complete freedom and flexibility. People with a *vata*-dominant *prakruti* are creative and free-spirited. They have amazing thinking power and perhaps a bent towards spirituality. They make talented artists, composers, writers, or scientists. Saraswati, the Vedic goddess of knowledge, personifies the inner beauty of the *vata dosha.* She is the consort of Brahma, the creator of the universe, and represents learning, creativity, knowledge, and vitality of the intellect. In mythology she is always depicted holding a veena (a wind instrument), a book, and a beaded necklace, each bead representing a branch of ancient Vedic knowledge. Physically, *vatas* tend to be small boned, with a tendency towards dry, thin, translucent skin; dry hair; cold extremities; and erratic eating patterns, behaviors, and habits. *Vatas* have a hard time sitting still.

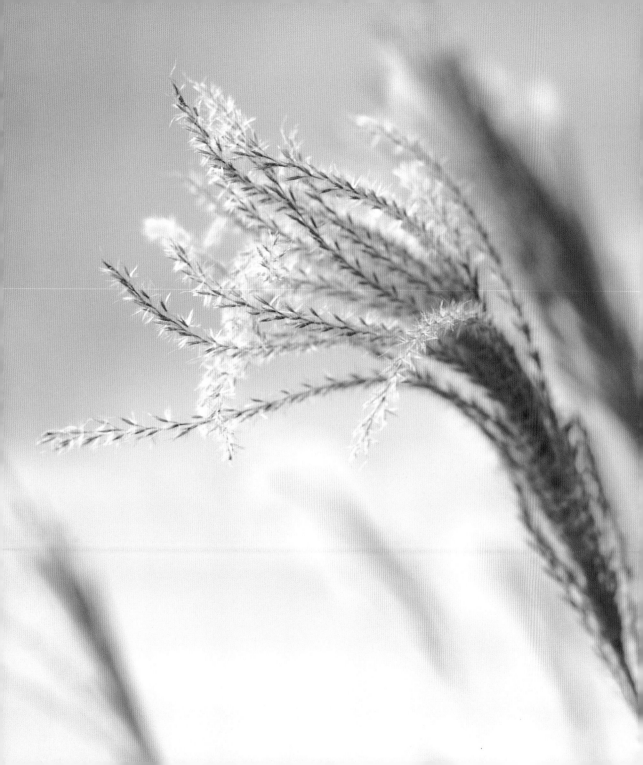

PITTA

The *pitta* constitution (fire and water) is like a volcano—it has a liquid heat smoldering deep inside, which sometimes accumulates and comes rushing out with dynamic intensity and drive. People with a *pitta*-dominant *prakruti* are intense, organized, and execution oriented, with a fantastic sense of purpose. They are able to process thoughts in a logical manner and make excellent leaders, managers, or mathematicians. Parvati (or Durga) is the goddess of strength and power, and well represents the beauty of the *pitta dosha*, which can at once be destructive and dangerous as well as powerful and seductive. She is the consort of Shiva, the destroyer of negativity, and is his counterpart in providing humanity with the power of active energy to choose good over evil, and so maximize *ojas*. Physically, *pittas* tend to have oily skin and hair with a "patchy" quality to it. (This can mean an uneven skin tone, combination skin that is more oily in the T-zone, thinner hair, and/or a certain flush to the skin.) Their hair and skin react easily to hormonal sensitivity and they are generally more prone to feeling hot and irritable.

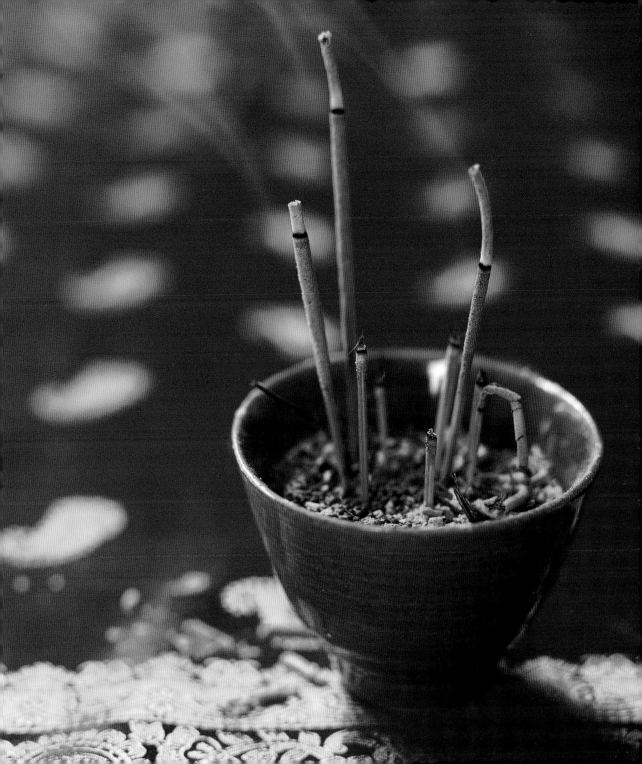

KAPHA

The soothing and stable qualities of *kapha* (water and earth) resemble those of clay—sand and water coming together to form something that can take shape and create vessels that have holding power without being easily disturbed. People with a *kapha*-dominated *prakruti* are nurturing, compassionate, meticulous, and have a wonderful ability to put physical structure to ideas and plans. These people make great health-care workers, caregivers, or workers in any occupation that requires persistence, physical stamina, and precision. Physically, they are heavier, stable people with skin that is cool and moist to the touch; thick hair all over the body; and thicker, more spongy skin. *Kaphas* tend to feel cold and break out into cool, clammy perspiration. The *kapha dosha* is synonomous with bounty and plentifulness, especially that which lasts a long time. Lakshmi, the goddess of wealth, exemplifies the beauty of the *kapha dosha*. The consort of Vishnu, the preserver of the universe, she is bountiful and earthy, always depicted with jewels and ornaments. Lakshmi is responsible for showering wealth and stability upon society, and exudes the golden luster of *ojas*.

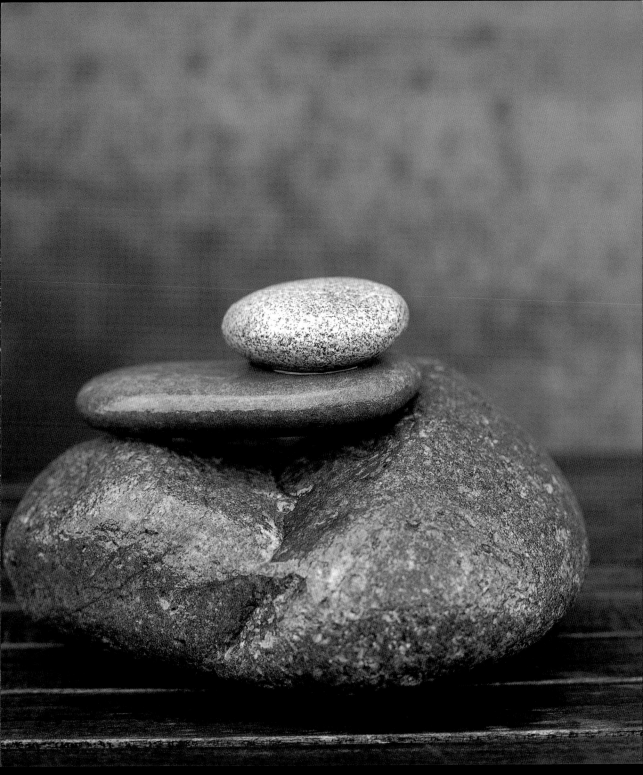

.:.:.:.:.:. DOSHAS THROUGH LIFE .:.:.:.:.:.

Each *dosha* is a type of energy that exists in the world around us, and each of these energies has a special influence on us during different stages of our lives. During childhood and youth, for example, *kapha* enhances chubbiness, so a plump baby is considered to have strong *ojas*. From puberty to menopause, *pitta* increases acidity and heat in the body, giving us the strength to carry us through those changes. Good stamina, leadership, and forbearance in transitional periods are all examples of strong *ojas* during the *pitta* phase of our lives. Later in life, *vata* predominates, bringing with it wrinkles, dry skin, and difficulty sleeping. But this is also the time in life when our spiritual abilities are at their highest potential. Wisdom and spirituality are examples of strong *ojas* during this life stage. For this reason, Indian women are generally more comfortable with their aging than Western women, and are also deeply respected by the people around them in their communities. Understanding your *prakruti* and how to increase your vitality will assure that you look and feel your best at every stage of life.

.:.:.:.:.:. DOSHAS OUT OF BALANCE .:.:.:.:.:.

When *doshas* go into a state of imbalance or excess, we experience low *ojas*. Imbalances *(vikruti)* refer to an excess, or accumulation, of any one or more of the *doshas*, causing negative forces and toxins to begin spreading through the body. Minor excesses of *vata*, *pitta*, or *kapha* are often manifested as dryness, a general sensation of heat, and heaviness in the mind and body. We often become hypersensitive and experience discomfort. For example, we may become intolerant of foods with similar *dosha* qualities as our predominant *dosha*. Left unattended, these imbalances can develop into illnesses, so it is important to be aware of their symptoms.

The pressures of modern life wreak havoc with our *doshas*. In ancient times, people modeled their lifestyle on nature and the seasons. Today, environmental influences like light, heat, and water that once ruled our work and sleep patterns now fall easily under our control. Conveniences like eating seasonal fruits year-round, driving instead of walking, and unhealthy diet and exercise habits distract us from our natural rhythms. As a result, it's easy to find yourself run-down, stressed, and feeling out of balance. Ayurveda recognizes the need to rejuvenate from within by setting the *dosha* composition back to *prakruti*, its natural starting point. This doesn't mean returning to the ways of our ancestors, but rather, gently adjusting our lifestyle to bring us back into balance.

Our predominant *dosha* is understandably the one most likely to become imbalanced. For example, *vatas* who are out of balance might have lower immunity and a tendency to catch colds on a regular basis. Each *dosha* expresses imbalance in a different way. Learning to read these signs will help you get back in balance quickly.

Vata is the most volatile of the three *doshas*. Too much *vata* energy creates dryness in the colon, causing pain, fatigue, and lowered immunity. It sets into the mind as anxiety, the inability to focus, and fear. People with *vata* imbalances tend to be "spacey" and forgetful. They lack the ability to focus and behave erratically. Low skin elasticity begins to manifest as wrinkles. This is exacerbated by delicate nerves and disturbed sleep patterns.

Pitta imbalances raise heat in the mid-digestive tract. Too much *pitta* energy manifests itself emotionally as anger, intolerance, and criticism or physically as acidity, inflammation, and sensitivities. People with *pitta* imbalances are prone to acne, heat toxins, any kind of "itis," food sensitivities (or allergies), cosmetics, dust, and pollen.

Kapha imbalances secrete excess juices in the upper digestive tract, causing sluggishness, depression, water retention, fat, and excessive mucus. People with too much *kapha* energy have clogged pores and follicles; mousy, congested skin; and manifest "couch-potato" behavior, where they remain lethargic and eat for comfort.

THE DOSHA QUIZ

This quiz will help give you a sense of your dominant *dosha*. While an Ayurvedic doctor or practitioner can most accurately determine your *prakruti,* this quiz will help you identify your primary *dosha,* the building block of your self-care routine. For each question, choose as many answers as you feel apply to you. All your answers do not have to be from the same *dosha* type. Rather than trying to answer based on how you feel right now, or want to look and feel, think specifically about how you usually look and feel. Whichever *dosha* you answer with the most often is your predominant *dosha*. Keep this *dosha* in mind as you read about the routines for personal care, yoga, and diet in the following chapters. While each of the *doshas* can go out of balance at any time, it is your dominant *dosha* that best predicts how you naturally feel. Over time, you can use this quiz again and again to see what your dominant *dosha* is in different phases of your life.

THE SKIN ON MY FACE IS . . .

VATA   normal to dry. I have fine lines and wrinkles. My skin lacks muscle tone or elasticity. It feels dry or tight when I travel, get dehydrated, or go out in cold weather.

PITTA   oily in the T-zone and dry on the cheeks. My skin tends to be sensitive and might redden or break out when exposed to chemicals, cosmetics, soap, and synthetics. I have many moles, freckles, or hyperpigmentation.

KAPHA   normal to oily. My skin tone is quite supple and elastic, although my face might get puffy. I have a tendency to have large pores and sometimes get whiteheads and pustules.

THE SKIN ON MY BODY IS . . .

VATA   normal to dry. It is thin and translucent, so you can often see my veins through the skin. It can lack elasticity and sag in some places. It might be rough or flake easily in certain areas.

PITTA   normal to sensitive. It has a warmth and a flush to it and reddens easily, especially in the sun or warmer climates. I might scar easily or have hyperpigmentation marks. I might also scratch my skin in response to sensitivities, which then causes my skin to scar.

KAPHA   normal, thick, and spongy. It has good, strong, supple tone and elasticity. My skin might retain water from time to time.

THE TEMPERATURE OF MY SKIN IS . . .

VATA   cool or cold. I have cold hands and feet, and I usually feel cold, especially in dry climates.

PITTA   warm. My skin is warm to the touch, especially in the upper torso, and my hands, feet, groin, and underarms tend to perspire. I feel hot and sweaty fairly readily, especially in warmer weather.

KAPHA   cold. My skin might even feel cool to the touch in fatty areas such as the buttocks, hips, thighs, or upper arms. My skin does not breathe well in cool, damp climates, and my pores tend to become clogged with oil. I often experience a cool, "clammy all over" kind of perspiration.

MY BODY FRAME IS . . .

VATA   small, lean, or wiry, either tall and thin or small and petite. I have lighter and less dense bones.

PITTA   compact, athletic, and muscular. I have a medium build and quite well-defined musculature and bone structure.

KAPHA   large. I have wide hips and shoulders. I have large muscles, and dense and heavy bones.

MY BODY FRAME HAS . . .

VATA   lesser amounts of fat right under the skin. I can lose (or gain) weight quite quickly and easily and can get "scrawny" at times.

PITTA   a medium layer of fat right under the skin (more in some areas and less in others). I have a good, strong metabolism and can gain or lose weight relatively easily.

KAPHA   thick layers of fat under the skin. I can gain weight easily, and find it relatively hard to lose weight.

WITHOUT CHEMICAL TREATMENTS, THE TEXTURE OF MY HAIR IS . . .

VATA   wavy, dry, with a flyaway tendency. My scalp tends to be dry and may flake when rubbed. I sometimes have dry scalp dandruff.

PITTA   fine, oilier in patches. My scalp can be sensitive to chemicals in hair products and prone to dandruff.

KAPHA   lustrous, beautiful, with natural shine and moisture. My scalp can be slightly oily to the touch. Sometimes the oil can clump up, forming large, oily dandruff.

THE STRENGTH AND THICKNESS OF MY HAIR IS . . .

VATA   inconsistent. While each individual hair might be thin and relatively dry or brittle, I have a lot of hair on my head.

PITTA   fine. Each individual hair is fine, and the overall volume is also fine, and can even seem scanty. I am prone to premature hair loss or graying hair.

KAPHA   thick. Each individual hair is strong, thick, and resistant to damage. I have lots of hair on my head.

MY NAILS ARE . . .

VATA   normal to dry. They break easily and are better managed if kept short. They might have ridges.

PITTA   pinkish and fairly strong.

KAPHA   big and thick with prominent white moons. They are strong and resistant to damage.

MY EYES ARE . . .

VATA   small with sparse lashes. They get dry easily and are sensitive to dust.

PITTA   sharp and clear. They are sensitive to bright light and redden easily with external influences like dust, pollen, cosmetics, strong light, or foods that do not agree with me.

KAPHA   large and picturesque, perhaps even dreamy. They might get puffy or have some whitish discharge from time to time.

MY DIGESTION IS . . .

VATA   irregular. Sometimes I'm hungry at mealtimes and sometimes I'm not. I might forget to eat and then feel spacey or weak, or tend towards constipation, gas, bad breath and hard, dry stools.

PITTA   intense. If I delay eating past my regular mealtimes, I get irritable. I sometimes have loose stools, heartburn, or acidity.

KAPHA   consistent or low. I can go without a meal if I am still full from the last one, but I also tend to eat for comfort. I often have a slower passage of thick, well-formed stools.

MY SLEEP PATTERNS ARE . . .

VATA   light and interrupted. I might stay awake for part of the night or have fitful, interrupted sleep. I usually can't remember my dreams, but when I do they tend to be vivid or imaginative.

PITTA   regular. I sleep about the same number of hours and feel rested. I have active dreams, sometimes even violent ones.

KAPHA   deep and heavy. I sleep long hours. I am not a morning person.

EMOTIONALLY SPEAKING, I AM . . .

VATA   quick-minded and imaginative. I am perceptive, excitable, and can get restless with creativity. I am friendly and exuberant.

PITTA   an organized and disciplined person. I am usually quite intense and passionate about what I do.

KAPHA   calm, steady, and nurturing. I do not get easily influenced or excited. I am a loyal, loving friend.

INTELLECTUALLY SPEAKING, I AM . . .

VATA   all over the place. I sometimes find it difficult to focus because I get excited about things. I tend to have a short memory.

PITTA   sharp, analytical, intelligent, and focused. I have a good memory, and good management and leadership skills.

KAPHA   a slower learner; I learn by doing and repetition. I have a long-term memory.

WHEN I MANIFEST EMOTIONAL IMBALANCES, I . . .

VATA   become anxious, stressed, nervous, or fearful.

PITTA   become critical, controlling, and angry.

KAPHA   become stubborn, stuck, and very hard to communicate with.

THE PACE OF MY LIFE IS . . .

VATA   intentionally fast. I keep myself busy to stay happy and prevent boredom.

PITTA   intense. My activities are well laid out and organized but require my absolute focus and involvement.

KAPHA   slow. I like to follow through my personal projects at my own pace.

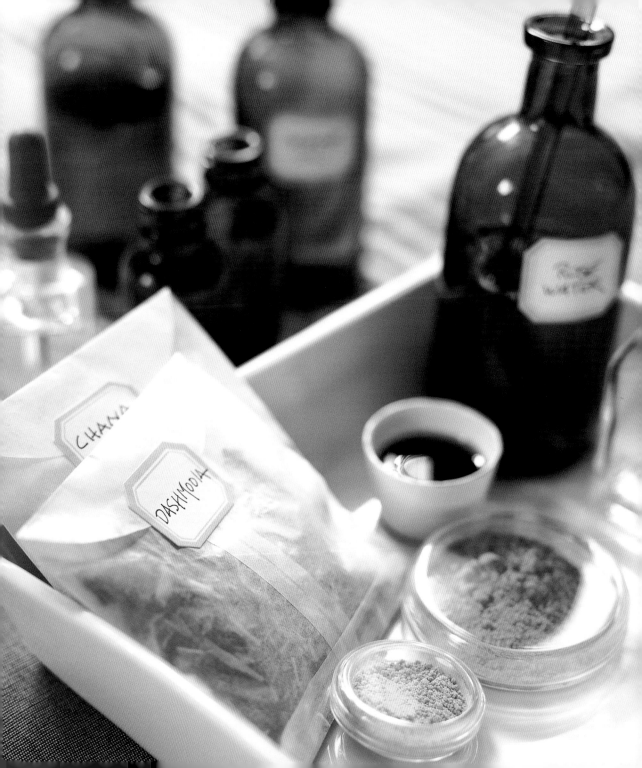

.:.:.:.:. **AYURVEDIC PANTRY** .:.:.:.:.:.

In the chapters that follow, the recommendations and recipes for self-care call for a number of ingredients, some common, some perhaps less familiar, and some that are probably completely new to you. This chart lists the staples of an Ayurvedic pantry and explains their significant properties for Ayurvedic practices. As you learn more about your *dosha* and the imbalances you tend to experience, you'll find yourself customizing this list to meet your personal needs.

Ayurvedic herbal ingredients are available through farmers' markets, natural-food stores, Indian stores, Ayurvedic stores, and mail-order suppliers (see Resources, page 139). Shop in places where you know the stock is turned over frequently, and use fresh herbs or whole-leaf dried herbs whenever possible. Dried herbs will begin to lose effectiveness after about six months, even sooner when ground, so only buy a little at a time. Some of these ingredients can be found in compounds such as *vata* tea, *pitta* tea, or *kapha* oil, so look out for them as you shop around.

OILS AND GHEE

COCONUT OIL	This cooling oil is ideal for balancing *pitta*. Used as both a hair and body oil, either alone or enhanced with medicinal herbs and flowers.
GHEE	Known in culinary terms as clarified butter, this is an ideal moisturizer for *vata*, as it is extremely penetrating, and *pitta*, as it is sweet and cooling. See also page 77.
MUSTARD OIL	This heating oil is ideal for *kaphas*. A common ingredient in cooking, it can be used as a moisturizer or in baths and *ubtans* (skin scrubs).
NEEM OIL	This anti-inflammatory and antiseptic oil is wonderful for cuts, abrasions, insect bites, and allergic reactions.
SESAME OIL	This warming, nutritious oil is suitable for all three *doshas*, and particularly for *vata*. It is used both in cooking and as a body moisturizer infused with medicinal herbs and flowers.

MEDICINAL HERBS

AMLA This fruit has a high content of Vitamin C and is full of antioxidants. It increases *ojas* in all tissues and is a powerful aid for balancing *pitta* in the blood cells and tissues.

BRAHMI Translated as "Divine Creative Energy," this rejuvenative herb, known to calm and cool the mind, is ideal for balancing *pitta* and *vata*. It is believed to promote intelligence and eternal youth and can be used in teas, salads, and hair oils.

DASHMOOL Meaning "ten valuables" in English, dashmool is a mixture containing the roots of ten key medicinal herbs. Ideal as an herb tea, this is a powerful ally in flu season.

NEEM The antiseptic quality of neem, a bitter herb celebrated for its blood-detoxifying and skin-healing properties, makes it a bitter yet extremely effective ingredient in cosmetics, medicinals, pharmaceuticals, and even tooth powders. It is used in *ubtans* to balance both *pitta* and *kapha*.

SANDALWOOD A *pitta*-balancing essential, sandalwood is used to rejuvenate and cool the skin. Applied to the forehead, it also takes the edge off headaches.

TRIPHALA The three fruits—amalaki, bhibhitaki, and haritaki—comprised in this mix balance each of the three *doshas* and cleanse the entire digestive system. Key to seasonal detox programs, triphala may be taken every day, as a tea with milk, or mixed with honey or ghee.

TULSI This plant, known as the "holy basil," has properties that aid in building immunity and preventing illness. Used in *ubtans*, in the bath, as an herb for tea, and in face packs, tulsi is an invaluable ingredient in skin care. Look for the fresh version at your local farmers' market, or purchase a plant for your home.

TURMERIC A powerful blood purifier, this common cooking spice is also a boon to *ubtan* formulas. Be careful to use only a small amount, as its color is quite penetrating and can stain the skin.

OTHER FOODS AND PLANTS

ALOE A cooling plant that grows in the hot desert terrain, this *pitta*-balancing gel is ideal both as a moisturizer and as a juice mix.

CHANA BESAN Also known as gram flour, this chickpea flour product is the perfect *ubtan* base. Used with turmeric root, sandalwood, tulsi, and other dried herbs to remove excess oil and cleanse the skin.

CUCUMBER Cooling and moisturizing, cucumbers are excellent for *ubtans* and moisturizers. Also use to cool hot, tired eyes.

GINGER An important Ayurvedic ingredient, this *vata*- and *kapha*-balancing root is useful for teas, oils, and food flavorings.

HEAVY WHIPPING CREAM
Highly nutritious and moisturizing, this is the perfect *vata*-balancing food for the mind, body, and skin.

HONEY A natural sweetner, ideal for tempering the challenging tastes of Ayurvedic medicinal herbs. As a humectant, it can also be added to any of the moisturizer recipes and is particularly ideal for the *vata* cleansers.

JASMINE Used for infusing in massage oils and baths for *vata* and *pitta;* the many varieties of this flower are quite fragrant. If the flower is not available, then an essential oil will do just as well.

ROSE WATER An ideal toner for all skin types; also an effective and gentle eye wash.

YOGURT Wonderful for balancing the pH of the skin, this is a widely used ingredient in *ubtans* and moisturizers.

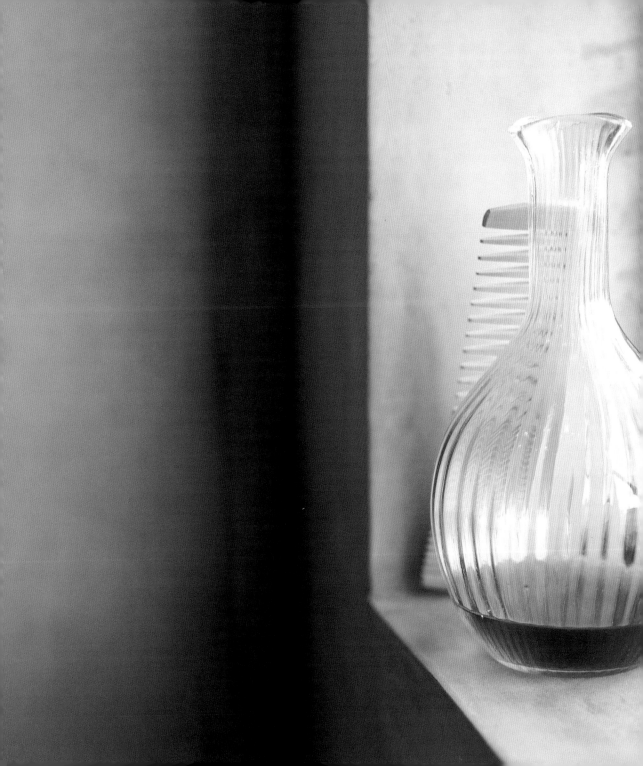

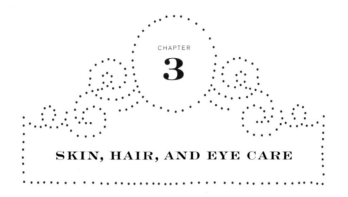

CHAPTER

3

SKIN, HAIR, AND EYE CARE

Ayurveda emphasizes beauty from within, a beauty that comes from health and well-being, not from cosmetics or anything that tries to cover up the true you. Because healthy skin and beauty go hand in hand, Indian women are encouraged to care for their complexions from a very young age. Simple, all-natural beauty treatments that emphasize balance and serenity have been passed down by Indian women from generation to generation. These easy routines for caring for your skin, hands and feet, hair, and eyes all help to balance the *doshas* and increase vitality, or *ojas*.

Since your face and body reflect your health and your feelings, the best way to look your best is to feel your best, by taking time out for yourself every day. The Ayurvedic daily routine (called *dinacharya*) is composed of a few simple rituals designed primarily to make you feel good. The daily regimen is as much a mind-set as it is a list of practices, and it includes things liking waking up early to maximize the day, cleansing, bathing, exercise, and a soothing, self-applied oil massage. Following these rituals allows us a few moments in the day to focus inwards, quiet our minds, and focus on appreciating the gift of health. While many of us feel like we do not have much time to take care of ourselves beyond a quick shower,

Ayurveda tells us that tending to our own minds and bodies with care is the starting point for living in harmony with the universe and contributing to the world around us.

.:.:.:.:. THE SKIN .:.:.:.:.

No matter how many times we hear or read that our skin is our biggest organ, many of us hang somewhere between forgetfulness and despair about our skin. Idealized perceptions of beautiful skin abound and can in turn intimidate; even the Vedic goddesses are referred to as having beautiful skin that has the radiance of sunshine and the smoothness of silk. Lakshmi, often described as beauty's bright goddess, is closely associated with Ayurvedic health and beauty—she was believed to have been born of Vishnu's churning an ocean of milk. For us mortals, Ayurveda teaches daily and weekly skin-care practices to make skin glow with inner and outer health. These focus on not only cleansing and protecting the skin but also stimulating and cleansing the blood and the lymph, the two primary fluids that directly feed the skin.

The Dosha Skin Types chart (right) will help you better understand your skin. Throughout this section, look for treatments appropriate to your skin type. If your skin is feeling normal, use any treatments for your *dosha* that appeal to you. If your skin is feeling unhealthy or showing signs of imbalance, enlist those treatments that target the problem: if dryness is your issue, for example, focus on moisturizing treatments that balance *vata*. You will also find self-massage techniques, simple bath soaks, and shower rubs for overall balancing.

DOSHA SKIN TYPES

Although by now you should have a good idea about which elements, or *doshas,* dominate in your constitution from taking the quiz in the previous chapter, it is worth taking a closer look at your skin specifically to see if it reflects one particular *dosha.* Regardless of skin type, many of us experience fluctuations in the mood of our skin from day to day and season to season. The following lists will help you determine your Ayurvedic skin type, what sensitivities to be aware of, and what signs of imbalance to watch out for.

VATA

COMPLEXION	Normal to dry, with a slightly rough texture
COLORING	Pale and thin, almost translucent, with veins sometimes showing through
PORES	Small, fine
SENSITIVITIES	Sensitive to changes in climate; tendency for chapping and dryness
AGING	Loses elasticity; tendency to sag and develop wrinkles and/or stretch marks
IMBALANCE	Excessive dryness or chapping (lips and skin); wrinkles or dark circles under the eyes, cellulite or stretched skin around the buttocks and thighs; peeling skin on feet and around toenails; corns and calluses

PITTA

COMPLEXION   Combination, oilier in the T-zone and drier on the cheeks; perhaps slightly oily to the touch

COLORING   Warm, soft, with strong coloring

PORES   Fine, with larger pores in the T-zone

SENSITIVITIES Sunburns easily, bruises easily, and tends to develop freckles, moles, or spider veins; sensitive to chemicals; tendency for blackheads and collecting sweat and dirt

AGING   Becomes sensitive with age, and prone to hot flashes

IMBALANCE   Excessive flushing, inflammation, acne, rosacea, hyperpigmentation; cold sores; athlete's foot or other fungal infections; easy scarring

KAPHA

COMPLEXION   Moist or oily to the touch; well toned, spongy or thick

COLORING   Cool, soft, with even coloring

PORES   Large all over

SENSITIVITIES Holds oil; tendency for whiteheads and clogged pores

AGING   Ages well, with maintained tone and minimal wrinkling

IMBALANCE   Swelling, water retention; clogged pores, whiteheads; puffy eyes; fatty lumps on the body; clammy hands, excessive oil and perspiration

.:.:.:.:.:. SELF-MASSAGE (ABHYANGA) .:.:.:.:.:.

Ayurvedic skin care begins with *abhyanga*, a therapeutic self-applied oil massage that nourishes the skin. Because looking good depends on feeling good, giving yourself a massage every day may be the best beauty secret we have. The combination of the gentle motion of the massage and the healing powers of herb-infused oils is optimum for stimulating the *dosha* energies to carry on their natural function and retain balance, as well as for toning the skin and its underlying muscles and tissue. The infused oils used for massage have rejuvenating properties that we miss out on if we think of all oils as impurities (like grease and dirt) or a source of automatic acne or other breakouts, since the right oils actually help remove toxins. Though Ayurvedic herbal extracts are available in creams, oils are much more effective moisturizers. If using oils feels strange to you, start practicing *abhyanga* with a light oil like almond or sunflower, and focus on the soothing effects of the massage. *Abhyanga* is traditionally a daily massage for the face and entire body, but if you do not have enough time for the full routine, focus on the head, face, hands, and feet for maximum results.

Ayurvedic self-massage is traditionally performed with oils prepared from medicinal herbs that balance the *doshas*. If you are feeling healthy, use the oil for your *dosha*, otherwise use the oil for the *dosha* that is out of balance (i.e., if your skin is irritated, use a *pitta* oil). While these herb-infused oils are available from specialty shops and from the resources listed in the back of this book, it is also easy to make your own simple infused oil by combining a base oil with readily available culinary herbs, spices, and flowers, many of which you might already have in your own kitchen. These oils will moisturize your skin gloriously while the scents transport your mind, and the massage you give yourself will give you time to focus inward every day. Here are some recipes for making your own Ayurvedic *abhyanga* oils. See the Ayurvedic Pantry on page 39 for more information on the ingredients used here.

ABHYANGA MASSAGE OIL

MAKES 1 CUP

VATA ABHYANGA OIL

    1 cup ghee or sesame base oil
    1/4 cup mixed herbs: turmeric-root powder, fresh ginger, lotus
        root, fresh basil, cloves, and fresh orange peel, in any
        combination
    Essential oils (optional): jasmine, basil, orange, rose

PITTA ABHYANGA OIL

    1 cup ghee, coconut, or sunflower base oil
    1/4 cup mixed herbs: turmeric-root powder, licorice root, and
        lemongrass, in any combination
    Essential oils (optional): saffron, sandalwood, coriander, lime

KAPHA ABHYANGA OIL

    1 cup canola or mustard base oil
    1/4 cup mixed herbs: turmeric-root powder, whole black pepper-
        corns, fresh ginger, fresh lemon peel, and cloves, in any
        combination
    Essential oils (optional): patchouli, lemon, eucalyptus, cardamom

1. In a small saucepan, heat the oil gently until it is beginning to boil but not smoking.
2. Stir in the herbs and remove from the heat.
3. Cover and let the herbs steep in the oil for 1 day or up to 2 days. Strain the oil through a coffee filter or a double layer of cheesecloth into an airtight container.
4. Add 5 to 8 drops of single or mixed essential oil, if desired.

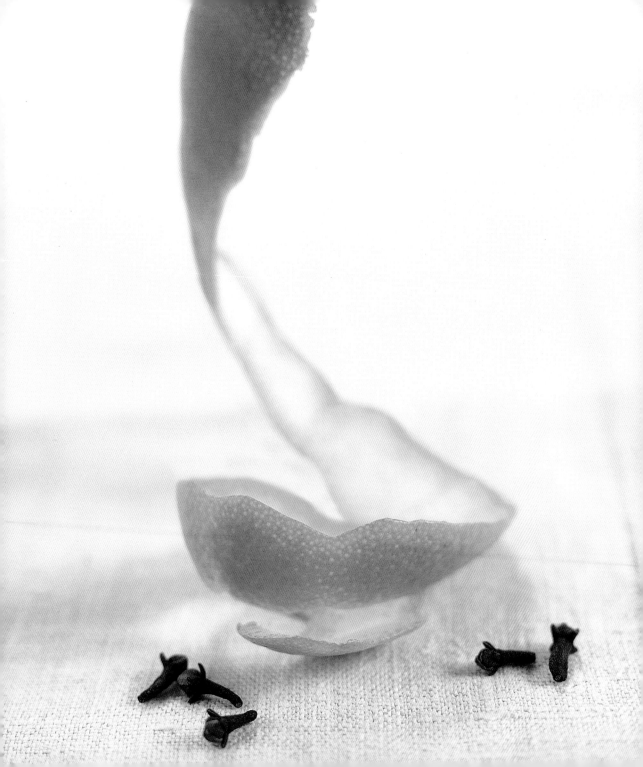

FULL-BODY ABHYANGA MASSAGE

Ayurvedic abhyanga *is traditionally done prior to bathing. Ideally, every morning you would spend 5 to 10 minutes on the massage routine, rest for about 15 minutes, then shower with a natural cleanser or nondetergent soap. If you don't have enough time in the mornings, rub in a light application of the oil following your shower, or aim to do it at night, after you shower and before you go to sleep.*

Abhyanga is worked from the center of the body outward to the extremities. This follows natural energy patterns, thus regulating tissue metabolism and providing for maximum distribution of ojas. Movements are either linear, following the layout of the muscles, or circular, applied typically to the joints, scalp, and vital energy points such as the navel. The linear movements encourage the natural flow of vata energy throughout the physical and emotional body; the circular movements help release energy in areas where it can become "stuck," leading to pitta or kapha imbalances. Heat your massage oil bain-marie style in a small bowl over warm water, or keep it at room temperature, if you like.

¼ to ½ cup *abhyanga* massage oil of your choice, homemade
   (page 48) or purchased

Pour a little oil onto the crown of your head and gently massage this area to help stimulate the release of heat and negative energy. Apply oil lightly and evenly all around your head and massage from the hairline to the crown, moving in small circles. Massage up and down the back of your neck. Massage in front of your ears, then behind, then your earlobes.

Rub your shoulders in small circles, then massage in straight lines from neck outward to shoulders. Massage from the center of your chest over the breastbone and out to your shoulders, then from the area where your ribs meet out to the periphery along and under the rib cage.

Placing one hand over the other, use your bottom hand to massage your navel in a small, clockwise circle (in the direction of the colon), and increase the size of the circle. Using both hands together (or placing one hand over the other for greater pressure), massage the front of your body from the navel to the left side of your waist, and up over your breast to the shoulder. Repeat on the other side, again using both hands. Use both hands to massage your waist from back to front.

Using the opposite hand, massage one shoulder in straight strokes down to the elbow and onto the hand. Rub the elbow and wrist in circles. Switch arms and repeat. Rub one palm, then the top of the hand. Pull and rotate each finger in succession. Massage the base of each finger. Switch hands and repeat.

Massage in straight strokes, as far as you can reach, from your lower back upwards. Use your left hand to massage the right shoulder blade up to the shoulder. Switch arms and repeat. Massage your hips and buttocks in outward circles, starting small and increasing the size of the circle as you go.

Massage the front and back of your thighs in straight strokes to the knees. Rub your knees in small, circular movements. Massage your calves from the knees to the ankles and back. Massage the ankles in vigorous, circular strokes. Massage the tops of your feet and the webs of your toes. Pull and rotate each toe in turn. Massage the balls of your feet. Rub the sole of one foot with the palm of the opposing hand to create friction. Repeat with the other foot.

ABHYANGA OF THE FACE AND NECK

Massaging your face and neck moisturizes the skin and also helps the abhyanga *oils to penetrate. Your massage movements should be applied up-wards, towards the temples, like a natural face-lift.*

2 to 3 tablespoons *abhyanga* oil of your choice, homemade (page 48) or purchased, warmed to room temperature if necessary

Apply oil lightly from the bridge of your nose over the cheeks and out to the ears. Rub your temples in small circles, then massage in circles up the hairline. Rub from the center of your eyebrows upward and outward over your forehead. Use three fingers of either hand to massage in circles all over your forehead.

Using both hands, massage in straight strokes from the center of your upper lip outward under the cheek bones to the ears. Using the index finger of each hand, rub over, around the inside edge, and then outside your nostrils in circular movements. Then use three fingers of each hand to massage in straight strokes outward from your nostrils to your ears. Massage in front of and around your ears. Massage your earlobes and inside the ears.

Apply gentle pressure on your cheekbones in an upward direction towards your temples. Pinch-press along your eyebrows, starting at the center of your brow and moving outward. Press on your eye sockets by closing your eyes and patting from the inside corners to the outside.

Starting with your fingers under your jaw, manipulate the area from your jawline to the base of your neck in a piano-playing motion, with gentle but firm pressure.

.:.:.:.:. BODY CLEANSING (UBTAN) .:.:.:.:.

In the Ayurvedic skin-care routine, *abhyanga* is followed with *ubtan*, a form of cleansing with therapeutic massage. *Ubtan* uses cleansing pastes prepared from herbs and flours or coarse grinds of legumes. These clarify the skin by drawing heat from the blood and stimulating lymph flow and also exfoliate the skin and firm the body. Traditional *ubtan* pastes use medicinal herbs such as manjishtha, neem, and sandalwood (see page 40) that break down congested toxins in the blood and lymph and encourage the body to shed toxins naturally. Babies are traditionally rubbed down with an *ubtan* paste at birth to cleanse them of impurities and strengthen their coordination.

Ubtan cleansers can be applied either as liquids, pastes, or powders, and are rubbed into the face and body fairly vigorously to stimulate the release of toxins. *Vata* types should use a liquid application with relatively large, circular movements; their skin being finer, powders can be a little too abrasive. *Pitta* types benefit from a paste application that can be easily worked in circular movements without overstimulating the skin. *Kapha* types require a powder application and should use small, vigorous, and vibratory circular movements to really stimulate the natural flow of body fluids. Remember that you can use the *ubtan* recipe for your *dosha*, or the *ubtan* recipe for the imbalance you are experiencing.

Ubtan cleansers are available in Ayurvedic shops and natural-products stores (see Resources, page 139), but following are some simple recipes for making your own. Make sure facial cleansers are ground smoothly enough not to irritate your skin. The facial cleansers may be used for the body as well. Because the skin of the body is less delicate than that of the face and neck, any cleanser used for the body can be coarser and used with a little more vigor to help tighten the pores and invigorate the underlying muscle and lymph tissue. When cleansing your body, if you have time, apply the *ubtan* paste and leave it on for 10 to 15 minutes until it begins to dry, then rub it off. See the Ayurvedic Pantry on page 39 for more information on ingredients used here.

FACIAL UBTANS

VATA FACIAL UBTAN

Vata *types benefit from a liquid* ubtan *that warms and moisturizes the skin.*

> 5 to 6 raw, blanched almonds, with skins removed
> 1/4 cup heavy whipping cream
> 2 tablespoons sesame oil
> 1 teaspoon brahmi or tulsi (see page 40)

1. In a bowl, soak the almonds in the cream overnight.
2. In a food processor, combine the almonds with the cream, the sesame oil, and the herb. Pulse until the mixture is smooth but yet has plenty of texture.
3. Rub into your face using gentle, circular motions.
4. Rinse off with cool to lukewarm water.

PITTA FACIAL UBTAN

This *pitta* ubtan *paste cools the skin and extracts heat toxins.*

> 3 teaspoons chickpea flour
> 1/4 teaspoon ground turmeric
> 2 teaspoons ground sandalwood or 1/2 teaspoon sandalwood
>   essential oil
> 1 teaspoon ground neem or neem oil (see page 39 and 40)
> 2 tablespoons crushed cucumber

1. In a bowl, stir together all the ingredients.
2. Rub the mixture into your face using small, circular motions.
3. Rinse with cool water.

KAPHA FACIAL UBTAN

Kapha *types benefit from a powdered* ubtan *that stimulates the skin to reduce water and accommodates natural lymph flow.*

> 3 teaspoons mung dal, or any variety of split peas (available in Indian shops)
> 1 teaspoon fenugreek seeds
> 1 teaspoon ground dried orange peel
> 1 teaspoon Ayurvedic herbs such as neem powder (see page 40), long (Pippali) pepper, or black pepper

1. With a mortar and pestle, crush all the ingredients, taking care to break up the mung dal into small pieces.
2. Rub the mixture into your face using small, vigorous circular movements.
3. Rinse with cold water.

UBTAN BODY SCRUB FOR ANY DOSHA

MAKES 1 FULL BODY APPLICATION

Here is a good, all-purpose tri-dosha ubtan *recipe for the whole body. Apply following your daily self-massage. Leave on for 10 to 15 minutes before rinsing, if you have time. Follow this with a light application of* abhyanga *oil to moisturize further.*

> 1 cup gram flour (available in Indian shops as chana besan)
> ½ teaspoon ground turmeric
> 2 tablespoons ground mustard
> 2 tablespoons crushed fresh coriander leaves
> 3 tablespoons rose water

For *vata dosha,* in a bowl combine all ingredients with ½ to ⅔ cup of ghee (see page 77) and stir to blend; mixture should be a relatively liquid paste. Smooth into the skin in gentle, circular movements, then rinse off with warm water.

For *pitta dosha,* in a bowl combine all ingredients with ½ cup orange juice and ½ cup water and stir to blend. Work into the skin vigorously, but without over-stimulating it.

For *kapha dosha,* in a bowl combine all ingredients with 1 cup yogurt and stir to blend; the mixture should be a relatively coarse paste. Work into wet skin vigorously, then rinse with warm water.

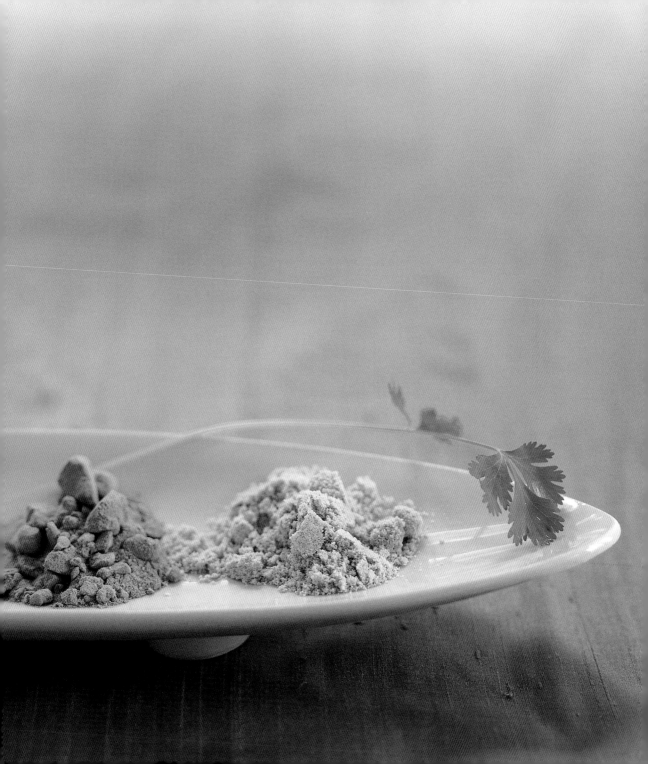

.:.:.:.:.:. BATHING .:.:.:.:.:.

In India, bathing represents a cleansing not only of the physical body but also of the spiritual self. Many purification rituals are associated with bathing; it is believed that ritual bathing in the waters of the Ganges River will purify the soul. In the simple Ayurvedic context, a bath taken in the morning following self-massage (see page 47) is likened to bathing in the Ganges.

In addition to cleansing body and spirit, bathing is also associated with numerous other benefits to the mind and body. The *Ashtanga Hridayam*, one of the ancient Ayurvedic texts, tells us that bathing improves sleep, appetite, sexual vigor, life span, and enthusiasm. The royal queens and princesses in ancient India were bathed in milk and fresh herbs to moisturize their skin until it glowed. To this day in India, special ingredients are stirred into a hot bath to customize it for *dosha*, time of year, or other considerations. For example, in the north, mustard is added to bath water in the winter months for a warm dip that balances *kapha dosha*, which can become aggravated in the late winter and early spring.

Bathing rituals are also believed to significantly impact health, especially over the long term. For example, warm water is believed to strengthen the body, while the face and head should be rinsed in cool water, as this is the area that naturally releases heat. Applying hot water to the head is believed to disturb the release of heat from the crown, thereby weakening the hair roots and encouraging emotional irritability and "hot-headedness." So while you can relax in a warm shower or bath, remember to wash your hair and face with cool water. Try the recipe below for your *dosha* for a balancing herbal cleansing bath. Remember that you can use the bath recipe for your *dosha*, or the one appropriate to any imbalance you are feeling. The mixtures can also be made with a little water or ground into a paste for use as a shower scrub.

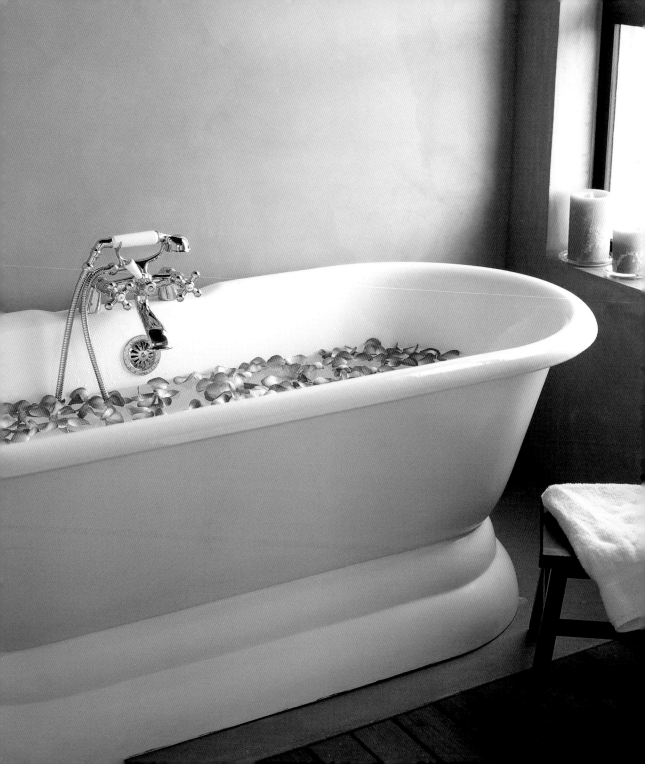

BATHS

VATA MILK AND RICE WATER BATH

The tradition of bathing in milk was begun by queens and noblewomen in ancient India. Milk contains proteins that are vital for nourishing the skin, and rice starch softens the skin and relieves stress. In a bowl, mix 1 cup powdered milk with 1 cup rice starch. Stir in 2 tablespoons of rose water for fragrance and softness. Dissolve the paste in your bath.

PITTA FRESH HERB AND FLOWER BATH

An herb and flower bath is perfect for soothing easily irritated *pitta*. You will be naturally perfumed with the fragrance of a Vedic garden. This is especially good in summertime, when *pitta* influence is at its peak. Add ½ cup marigold, rose, or jasmine flower petals and a handful of cooling fresh herbs such as mint or coriander to your bath water. Adding a couple of tablespoons of lemon juice or white vinegar will help balance excess oil and get rid of blemishes.

KAPHA MUSTARD AND FENUGREEK BATH

This combination of herbs is traditional in the cold winter and winter monsoon season of the Punjab region. Use year-round, but especially during the late winter and through spring, when *kapha* influence is at its peak. Add 3 table-spoonfuls ground mustard and 1 tablespoon fenugreek powder to your bath.

Moisturizing the skin is extremely important to alleviate drying *vata* tendencies and to maintain suppleness and elasticity. The use of natural
foods, botanicals, and oils are the traditional Ayurvedic approach to nourishing and replenishing the skin. Moisturizing the face and neck can be
done in the morning or in the evening, but is a must for your everyday routine *(dinacharya)*. (Moisturizing the entire body is undertaken once a
week; see page 64.) *Vata* types with drier skin would do well to moisturize
face and neck twice a day, whereas *pitta* and *kapha* types can get away with
moisturizing just once a day.

Below you'll find moisturizer recipes for each *dosha*; remember
that you can use the recipe for your *dosha*, or one that matches any imbalances you are experiencing. Since Ayurvedic moisturizers are made from
natural ingredients that can grow bacteria, they do not keep too long.
Prepare enough to last 1 week at a time, ¹/₂ to 1 cup, and store in a cool, dry
place. Avoid refrigerating the moisturizers, though, as this will disrupt the
natural chemistry with your skin in relation to the climate or outside temperature.

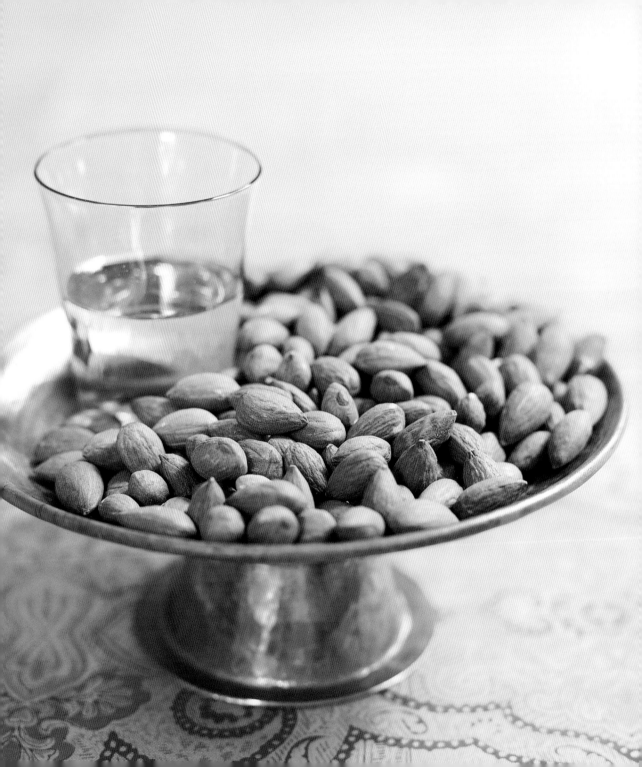

MOISTURIZERS

VATA

Vata skin needs plenty of natural moisture and oil to keep it supple and maintain elasticity. Ghee (see page 77) is one of the best moisturizer bases for *vata* skin. In a bowl, mix together equal parts ghee and rose water. Add a teaspoon of honey and few drops of your favorite essential oil to add fragrance. Transfer to a jar with a tight-fitting lid. Rub a small amount of the solution onto your face and neck at least once a day. This recipe makes an ideal moisturizer for both day and night applications for *vata* skin types. Sesame oil may be substituted for ghee.

PITTA

Pitta skin needs a light moisturizer that is also cooling. Aloe is an ideal ingredient for both moisture and the wonderful soothing sensation it brings. For a daytime moisturizer, in a bowl, combine 1 part brewed licorice tea, 1 part aloe vera gel, and 2 parts coconut or sunflower oil. Use the moisturizer on your face and neck at least once a day. At night, moisturize with equal parts aloe and ghee, or just plain ghee.

KAPHA

Kapha skin is generally well toned and needs only a mild balancing moisturizer. Pure mustard oil is an ideal base. In a bowl, mix together equal parts mustard oil and almond oil. Add a few drops of your favorite essential oil to help dissipate the strong smell of mustard. This moisturizer is ideal for head-to-toe use, both day and night, but if the faint smell of mustard during the day bothers you, almond or sunflower oils are good alternatives for *kapha* skin.

WEEKLY SKIN-CARE RITUALS

Beyond your daily skin-care regimen, it is a good idea to establish a weekly skin-care ritual—a guaranteed time-out will truly work to beautify from within. While the guidelines outlined previously address your "must do" self-care for every day *(dinacharya)*, we need to go a little beyond this to really work at pulling out toxins and maintaining balance for maximum *ojas* through the year. Traditionally many of these inner-beauty routines were followed as part of a daily detox and self-care program, but these days, our busy schedules and work or family commitments do not allow for deeper self-care on an everyday basis, so it's practical to seek out a routine that we can perform at least once a week. Try the weekly ritual ideal for your *dosha* described on the following pages, or switch to those for other *doshas* when you are feeling imbalanced. The most important part of the experience is to focus inward and tune into the needs of your *dosha.* As you incorporate a weekly cleansing into your lifestyle, you should over the weeks begin to perceive a positive difference in your emotional being as you work from the angle of your physical being. See the Ayurvedic Pantry on page 39 for more information on the ingredients used here.

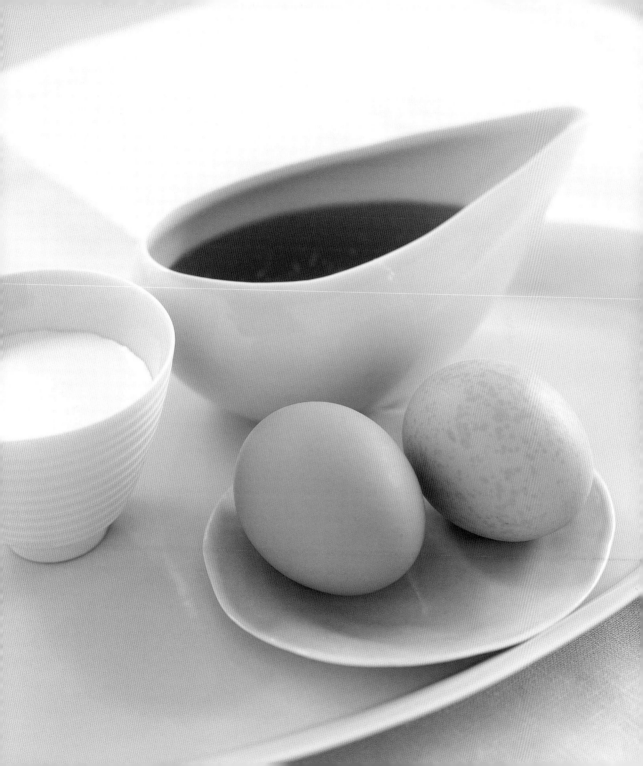

WEEKLY CLEANSING MASKS

VATA WEEKLY CLEANSING MASK

1 egg white
1 teaspoon honey
1 teaspoon rose water
1 cup plus 2 teaspoons heavy whipping cream

Following self-massage (see page 47), prepare a mask by whisking together the egg white, honey, rose water, and the 2 teaspoons cream in a bowl. Set aside.

Prepare a steam bath by turning on a hot shower and letting it run for a few minutes until it begins to generate steam. Point the showerhead away from you so that you can step into the shower cubicle or tub to immerse yourself in the steam, but without actually getting wet from the running water, if possible, or clear a space outside the tub or shower where steam is accumulating. Remove all of your clothing and enter the steamy area, closing the shower curtain or door if applicable so that the steam does not escape. Find a place to sit if there's not a natural perch—if there is room, position a chair in the space. Rest in the steam bath for about 10 minutes. Turn off the shower.

Apply the mask to your face and neck. Step into the tub or shower area if you are not already there and leave the mask on for 15 minutes while rubbing the 1 cup cream all over your body. You should be able to stay warm from all of the steam that has been generated.

Rinse your face and body thoroughly; your skin will feel soft and supple.

PITTA WEEKLY CLEANSING MASK

  2 teaspoons sandalwood powder
  Pinch of ground turmeric
  1 teaspoon neem oil (see page 39)
  2 tablespoons natural clay (available at health-food stores)
  ¼ cup fresh orange juice
  1 cucumber, peeled and coarsely crushed
  2 teaspoons ground neem (see page 40) or fresh coriander leaves
  or seeds

Following self-massage (see page 47), prepare a mask by stirring together the sandalwood, turmeric, neem oil, clay, and orange juice. Set aside.

Separately, stir together the cucumber and ground neem or coriander.

Prepare a steam bath by turning on a hot shower and letting it run for a few minutes until it begins to generate steam. Point the showerhead away from you so that you can step into the shower cubicle or tub to immerse yourself in the steam, but without actually getting wet from the running water if possible, or clear a space outside the tub or shower where steam is accumulating. Remove all of your clothing and enter the steamy area, closing the shower curtain or door if applicable so that the steam does not escape. Find a place to sit if there is not a natural perch—if there is room, insert a chair in the space. Rest in the steam bath for about 5 minutes. Turn off the shower.

Apply the mask to your face and neck. Step into the tub or shower area if you are not already there and leave the mask on for 15 minutes while rubbing the cucumber mixture all over your body.

Rinse your face and body thoroughly; your skin will feel both deeply cleansed and moisturized.

KAPHA WEEKLY CLEANSING MASK

    2 teaspoons ground neem (see page 40)
    Pinch of ground turmeric
    2 tablespoons natural clay (available at health-food stores)
    4 teaspoons plus 2 tablespoons ginger juice
    1 cup yogurt
    2 tablespoons salt
    2 tablespoons ground black pepper

Following self-massage (see page 47), prepare a mask by stirring together the ground neem, turmeric, clay, and 4 teaspoons ginger juice.

Separately, stir together the yogurt, salt, pepper, and the 2 tablespoons ginger juice. Set aside.

Prepare a steam bath by turning on a hot shower and letting it run for a few minutes until it begins to generate steam. Point the showerhead away from you so that you can step into the shower cubicle or tub to immerse yourself in the steam, but without actually getting wet from the running water if possible, or clear a space outside the tub or shower where steam is accumulating. Remove all of your clothing and enter the steamy area, closing the shower curtain or door if applicable so that the steam does not escape. Find a place to sit if there is not a natural perch—if there is room, insert a chair in the space.

Apply the mask to your face and neck. Step into the tub or shower area if you are not already there and leave the mask on for 15 minutes while rubbing the yogurt mixture all over your body. You should be able to stay warm from all of the steam that has been generated.

Rinse your face and body; your skin will feel toned and detoxified.

Bathing and skin care for your hands and feet deserve a special note. Ayurveda honors the hands and feet, and considers them magnets that attract life energy. Vedic goddesses are portrayed with multiple arms and hands holding symbolic objects or positioned in poses called *mudras* that instill divine energy. Walking in bare feet is thought to draw energy from the earth. Washing and massaging the hands and feet every day is therefore an essential part of Ayurvedic self-care. Massaging the hands and feet boosts circulation, helping alleviate *vata* problems like dryness or cold extremities, as well as *kapha* problems such as water retention.

The hands and feet reveal much about any *dosha* imbalances we are suffering. Use the chart below to identify constitutional imbalances, and read on for the solutions that are best for you.

VATA	Wrinkled or rough hands
	Rough, hard feet
	Nails that break or peel easily or have ridges
	Cold hands and feet
PITTA	Fungus in the nails
	Athlete's foot
	Cuticles that bleed easily
	Hot, sweaty hands and feet
KAPHA	Puffy, swollen hands
	Cold, clammy hands and feet
	Thick layers of superfluous skin
	Heavy, clumsy movement of the extremities

As a general practice, wash hands and feet with a mild soap, and then massage with the appropriate Ayurvedic *abhyanga* oil to relieve *dosha* imbalances. Or, for simple, all-purpose moisturizing, use sesame oil or ghee (see page 77).

Once a week, give your hands and feet a balancing treatment with a special scrub and moisturizer. You'll be amazed how smooth and supple your skin feels, resonating with the vital energy of the earth.

For *vata* and *kapha* imbalances, make a paste of 1 teaspoon rock salt, ½ teaspoon ground cloves, and 2 tablespoons sesame oil. Rub the mixture in small circles into both hands and feet, focusing on the heels, soles, ankles, finger and toe webs, fingers and toes, wrists, and palms.

For *pitta* tendencies, make a solution of 1 teaspoon neem oil (see page 39) and 2 tablespoons coconut oil and massage into both hands and feet, focusing on the heels, soles, ankles, finger and toe webs, wrists, and palms.

For an all-purpose treatment, rinse the hands and feet with the juice of 1 lemon diluted in 1 cup of warm water. Dry off with a soft, fluffy towel. Finish off by massaging 3 to 5 tablespoons of heavy whipping cream into your hands and feet to moisturize thoroughly.

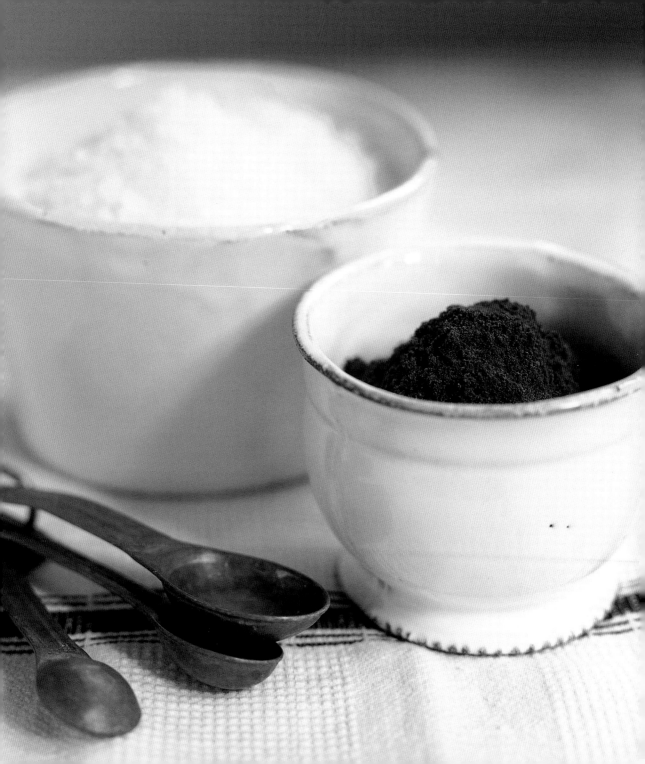

.:.:.:.:. HAIR .:.:.:.:.

In India, hair symbolizes strength for men and beauty for women. It is believed that the Ganges, the holy river of India, was released to the earth through Lord Shiva's tresses. Because of the belief that a significant amount of strength lies within the hair, Ayurveda prescribes everything possible to keep a cool head and maximize hair thickness. Internal heat is expelled through the top of the head, and higher levels of internal heat correspond to less hair, which is why *pitta* types tend to have thinner hair than *kapha* and *vata* types. Ayurvedic beauty rituals for the hair and scalp use cooling oils and other *pitta*-balancing herbs, fruits, nuts, and flowers that focus on removing heat, strengthening hair follicles, and promoting thickness. Yoga, *pranayama*, and *abhyanga* techniques also focus on releasing heat through the crown.

Basic imbalances in the *doshas* can lead to problems of the hair and scalp. *Vata* imbalances (and also hair dryers) can cause dry, brittle, or flyaway hair and dandruff. *Pitta* imbalances cause itchiness in the scalp or premature graying and hair loss. *Kapha* imbalances dull the hair and scalp with excess oil secretions, which sometimes result in large flakes of oily dandruff.

Ayurvedic hair care is much more gentle than that of the West. Hair is not washed every day; daily cleansing strips the scalp of natural oils and encourages the sebaceous glands to produce more oil than necessary. Instead of washing the hair often and then using multiple products to restore shine and softness, hair is conditioned with oil prior to limited shampooing.

Begin your practice of Ayurvedic hair care by learning to brush your hair thoroughly every day, and wash it only once or twice a week. (This can be hard to get used to at first, but you'll soon find that washing your hair less often rebalances the flow of natural oils to your scalp, making it shiny and well conditioned.) Then adopt the hair-care basics detailed below for strong and beautiful hair for any *dosha*.

ARITHA SHAMPOO

MAKES 1 APPLICATION

Aritha, the fruit of the soapnut tree, is extremely gentle and is an effective agent for cleaning your hair without stripping the natural oils (though it will not lather like regular shampoos). Shikakai, another Ayurvedic botanical, provides additional conditioning. Both are commonly available at Indian stores (or see Resources, page 139.)

  1 cup whole aritha nuts or ½ cup aritha powder
  2 tablespoons shikakai powder
  1 tablespoon fresh lemon juice

Soak the aritha nuts in 1 cup of water overnight. (If using aritha powder, just stir into 1 cup water and proceed with adding the lemon juice.) Strain the soaking liquid through a coffee filter or cheesecloth and add the shikakai powder and the lemon juice. Apply the entire amount to your hair (be careful not to get the mixture into your eyes as the aritha will sting) and rinse with cold water. It is best to let your hair air-dry, although you can blow-dry and style it as you are accustomed to, if necessary. (If you can't find aritha, add 1 tablespoon of all-purpose Ayurvedic hair oil or plain coconut oil to your regular shampoo for additional conditioning.)

COCONUT AND FLOWER HAIR OIL

MAKES 1 APPLICATION

Oiling your hair is the most important part of Ayurvedic hair care. Not only does it beautify the hair and scalp, it helps to reduce heat from the head, thus promoting sleep, relaxation, and memory and increasing your all-around vitality, or ojas. Use this basic oil to condition your hair before shampooing, or, if you like, purchase the traditional Ayurvedic oils that contain bhringhraj, brahmi, or amla at an Ayurvedic store.

½ cup coconut oil
2 tablespoons rose water
½ cup mixed fresh flower petals such as hibiscus, marigold, rose, or jasmine

1. In a small saucepan, bring the oil to a boil.
2. Add the rose water and flowers, return to a boil, and cook for 3 minutes.
3. Remove from the heat.
4. Let the flowers steep in the oil for 1 day, then strain the oil through a coffee filter or a double layer of cheesecloth into an airtight container.

To oil your hair, gently massage 4 to 5 tablespoons of the oil onto the crown of your head and into your scalp. Comb the oil out to the ends of the hair. You can apply a turban made from a towel or plastic wrap so the oil really penetrates. Leave the oil on for at least 20 minutes, or up to overnight.

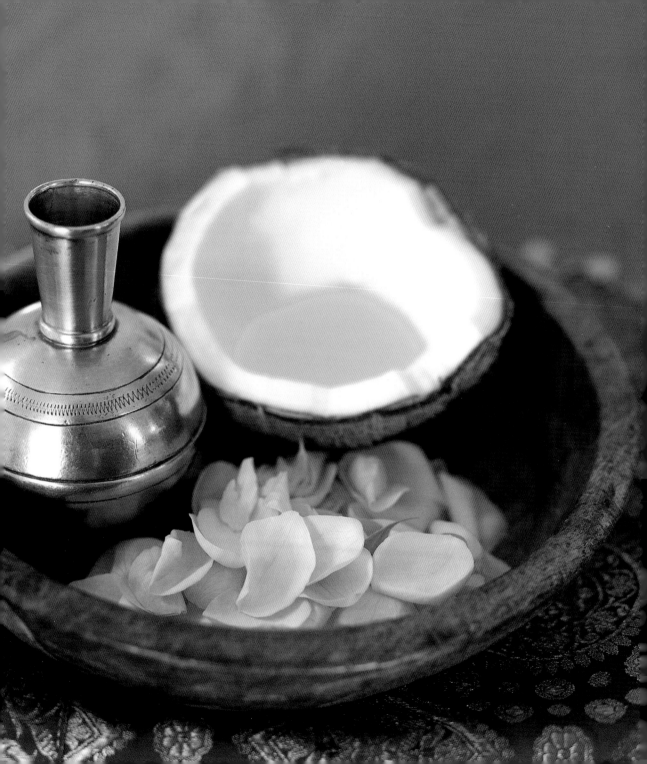

In Indian tradition, eyes radiate powerful energy—just look at any painting of the goddesses' almond-shaped eyes. Keeping the eyes healthy is the best way to keep their powers at their peak—not to mention the best way to discourage dark circles, fine lines, and red, itchy, watery eyes. The Ayurvedic approach to caring for the eye area is unique because it takes into account the eye itself, the skin around the eye, and even how what you see affects you. Moisturizing your lids and caring for the surface of your eyeballs as well as gazing upon something beautiful are equally important ways of caring for your eye area.

The eyes are delicate and susceptible to various imbalances of the *doshas.* Sudden changes in temperature, straining, excessive crying, feeling angry, suppressing emotions, pollution, and intoxicants all harm the eyes. *Vata* imbalances dry out the eyes, causing wrinkles, lines, and crow's-feet and twitching eyelids. *Pitta* eyes can become itchy, red, heated, and sensitive to light. *Kapha* imbalances lead to eye puffiness, swelling, and perhaps excess secretion or glazed vision.

To keep your eyes healthy, wash your eyes with cool water or rose water every morning, being sure to open your eyes for ablution. Once a week, apply 3 to 5 drops of ghee (see facing page) to the eyes to keep them cool. Or wash your eyes with ghee using an eyecup, filling the entire eyecup with ghee and placing it over one eye. Slowly open your eye to the ghee in the cup and blink and rotate your eyeball to bathe completely. When you are done with the ghee eye bath or application of ghee drops, gently massage the skin under and around the eyes with a little more ghee or a few drops of heavy whipping cream. To complete the ritual, pinch the eyebrows from inside to outside and apply gentle pressure on the eye socket from inside to outside.

GHEE—THE LONGEVITY ENHANCER

Ghee, or clarified butter, is believed in Ayurveda to be one of the most sattwic *foods, as it promotes memory, intelligence,* agni *(digestive fire), and* ojas. *Excellent for all three* doshas, *though specifically for* vata *and* pitta, *ghee is ideal for cooking, as it has a high smoke point and does not burn easily. It provides nourishment to the body and builds healthy tissue when used in cooking, when taken alone, or when prepared with medicinal herbs for skin, scalp, and eye treatments. Ghee is also used for* abhyanga.

Although ghee is readily available at Indian grocery stores, it is simple to make your own. Clean and sterilize a saucepan by filling it with water, covering it with the lid, and bringing it to boil for 30 minutes. Discard the water and add 1 pound of unsalted organic butter cut into chunks to the pan and heat over low heat for 10 to 15 minutes, until the foam that collects on the surface begins to settle on the bottom of the pan. Continue to cook, stirring occasionally, until the ghee begins to boil gently. Remove from the heat and let cool. Pour off the clarified butter on top into a clean container, leaving the sediment at the bottom of the pan. As long as it is kept away from moisture and other contaminants, ghee keeps indefinitely without refrigeration because all the milk fats that cause butter to spoil have been removed.

When ghee is at room temperature, it can be semisolid, so run warm water over the closed container to soften it before use in treatments.

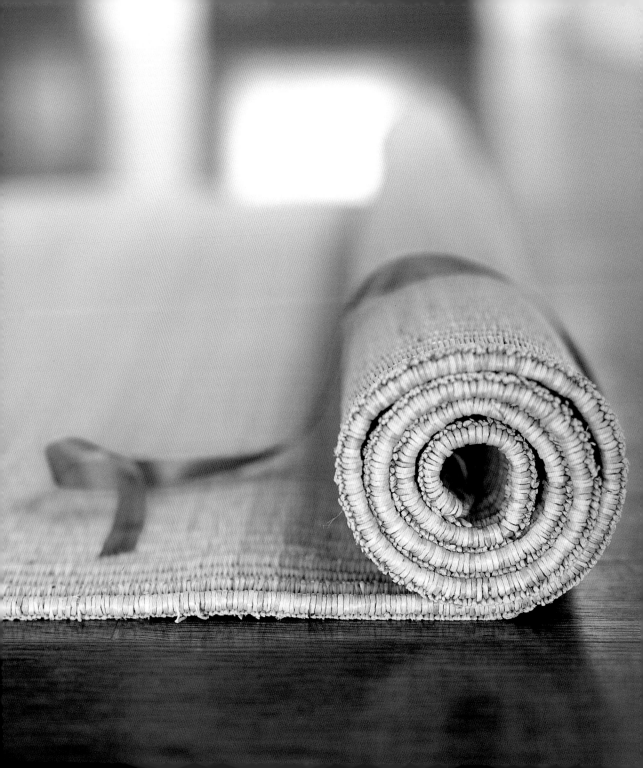

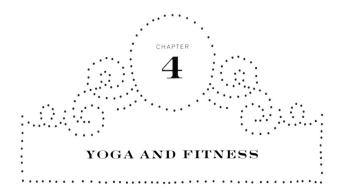

CHAPTER

4

YOGA AND FITNESS

A tranquil mind and body, free of stress and tension, is the ultimate beauty secret. Exercise creates vitality, called *ojas* in Ayurveda, by releasing stress and building strength, flexibility, and increased stamina. The results: glowing skin, a good mood, and a new sense of serenity. While every kind of exercise has its particular benefits, yoga is the perfect complement to Ayurveda because its ultimate purpose is to regularize the flow of vital energy, or *prana*, in the system to increase *ojas*.

Yoga means "union," as in that of the mind, body, and breath. This integrated approach makes yoga very different from other forms of exercise. For example, instead of developing our voluntary muscles to their greatest capacity, yoga works with breath and movement to help us gain control of our internal organs and involuntary muscles. Instead of working the body to a point where it needs to rest in order to rejuvenate and strengthen itself, yoga invigorates the body by using the breath in a way that creates inner strength and stamina. In particular, the Ayurvedic approach to yoga includes cleansing of the mind and thoughts in order to detoxify the system—this is considered as important to the workout as your arms and legs. Ayurveda encourages various traditions of yoga, although the Hatha yoga tradition is the easiest to follow as a self-care technique. An Ayurvedic approach to yoga goes beyond the physical postures (asanas) to include meditative breathing *(pranayama)*, massage *(abhyanga)*, and cleansing rituals to awaken the body and control the subtle heating and cooling energies that we experience in yoga.

Yoga and Ayurveda are sister disciplines. The original texts of yoga and Ayurveda were both written by the snake bearer of the Hindu god Lord Vishnu, the preserver of the universe, during his earthly incarnation. In this context, "preservation" means those actions that sustain and develop human life. Ayurveda and yoga both preserve the physical, emotional, and spiritual body by simple self-care through daily life. Yoga believes that you are as young as you are flexible, and emphasizes the development of flexibility along with breath control to promote longevity.

.:.:.:.:. **YOGA STYLES** .:.:.:.:.:.

Many styles of yoga have developed over the last several years. The differences lie in emphasis, such as focusing on strict alignment of the body, coordination of breath and movement, holding the postures, or the flow from one posture to another. All of the styles share a common lineage and are based on Patanjali's *Yoga Sutras,* the classical yoga texts of ancient India. No one style is "better" than another, although certain styles are favorable to particular *doshas.* Above all, it is important to find a style that you are comfortable with and a teacher that you can trust to improve your yoga practice.

HATHAYOGA

Hathayoga is a classical style of yoga that is described in the Yoga sutras and that forms a base for many styles of yoga. It uses poses (asanas), breathing *(pranayama)*, and relaxation to awaken, experience, and control the subtle energies within oneself. It provides strength and flexibility through a relatively gentle, inward experience.

ASHTANGA

Ashtanga yoga is physically demanding. You flow through a series of poses, jumping from one posture to another to build strength, flexibility, and stamina. "Power yoga" is based on Ashtanga.

BIKRAM

Bikram yoga comprises a series of twenty-six asanas performed in a heated room. The routine is designed to warm and stretch muscles, ligaments, and tendons in the order in which they should be stretched. Many asanas are performed twice and then held to build intensity.

INTEGRAL

Integral yoga puts a good deal of emphasis on breathing and meditation in addition to postures. This is a consciousness-oriented yoga that emphasizes healing and transformation. Integral yoga is used by Dr. Dean Ornish in his groundbreaking work on reversing heart disease.

IYENGAR

Iyengar yoga is one of the most popular styles of yoga in the world. Its great attention to detail and the precise alignment of postures is aided by the use of props such as blocks and belts. The sequences are systematized by level and can be gentle or challenging.

KRIPALU

Kripalu yoga is often called the "yoga of consciousness." It emphasizes proper breath, alignment, and coordinating breath and movement, working according to the limits of your individual flexibility and strength. You learn to focus on the physical and psychological reactions caused by various postures to develop an awareness of mind, body, emotion, and spirit.

KUNDALINI

Kundalini yoga focuses on the controlled release of *kundalini*, a powerful energy that is believed to be seated at the base of the spine. The practice involves classic poses, breath, coordination of breath and movement, and meditation to release this energy upwards through the spine.

VINIYOGA

Viniyoga develops practices for individual conditions and purposes. Asanas integrate the flow of breath with movement of the spine, and include sequencing, intensity adaptations based upon the overall goals. Function is stressed over form.

.:.:.:.:. **YOGA FOR YOUR DOSHA** .:.:.:.:.

VATA	Hathayoga, Bikram, Viniyoga, Kripalu
PITTA	Iyengar, Viniyoga, Kundalini, Integral
KAPHA	Ashtanga, Bikram, Viniyoga, Kundalini

TRADITIONAL NASAL CLEANSING

JALNETI

The Ayurvedic tradition of *jalneti* is the act of clearing the nasal passages with herb-infused water. Although it may seem hard or uncomfortable, with a little practice it's easy to do, and highly effective. Allergy sufferers will particularly benefit from this practice, as cleansing the nasal passages with water and herbal oils purifies the system and helps regulate pressure in the head. It is best practiced in the morning prior to breath exercises such as *pranayama*. *Jalneti* is traditionally performed with a small pot called a neti pot that looks like a miniature teapot with a particularly long spout (see Resources, page 139). Fill the neti pot with about 1 cup of lukewarm water. Add 5 to 7 drops of an herbal essential oil or other concentrate that brings out toxins and relieves congestion (if these are not available, a teaspoon of table salt will help break down the upper levels of congestion). Place the spout at the right nostril (but do not insert into the nostril), keeping your mouth open to allow for free breathing, and tip the pot to send the water into your right nostril. Tilt your head slightly forwards and to the left so that the water flushes through the nasal passages and emerges from your left nostril by the force of gravity. This is going to feel strange at first! Should any nasal congestion prevent the free flow of water, allow some time to elapse before trying again. When the pot is empty, refill and repeat with the other nostril. Work up to 2 potfuls per day on each side. Nasal cleansing is good for all three *doshas*.

.:.:.:.:. YOGA DINACHARYA—YOGA RITUALS FOR EVERY DAY .:.:.:.:.

While many treat yoga as an outlet for physical exercise, there's really more to it than just the poses, or asanas. Without incorporating the other aspects of yoga, according to the ancient texts, it is nearly impossible to get the maximum benefits out of the physical postures. While you may feel like you don't have time in your life right now to do a full practice all the time, start by making time when you can; you may discover it's an easier habit to cultivate than you think. Even enjoyed only once in a while, yoga is a great restorative when you really need to take care of yourself. A full yoga practice is ideally done in the mornings, although it may be done in the evenings as well.

A complete yoga practice has five parts. First, perform a simple self-massage (abhyanga), as described on page 47. Second, try the nasal cleansing routine to detoxify the system, as described on page 83. Third, using the guide below, develop a routine of yoga postures that are suited to your dosha-balancing objective, or attend your favorite yoga class. Fourth, end your workout by taking time for an exercise to control and focus the breath. Lastly, meditate on a favorite image, situation, or positive thought.

.:.:.:.:. YOGA TO BALANCE YOUR DOSHA .:.:.:.:.

While working with an experienced yoga instructor is optimum for truly tailoring yoga for Ayurvedic needs, it is easy to incorporate dosha-aware-ness into your practice at home. Following are simple yoga routines for each dosha that can help correct imbalances, or vikruti, on a day-to-day basis. Each sequence starts gently and builds in intensity as it goes along. Remember, you do not necessarily have to do the entire sequence every day. Depending on your dosha, your health on a particular day, and your goals, your yoga can be a gentle, inward experience, or an athletic or aerobic practice.

VATA YOGA ROUTINE

Vata imbalances generally mean you're not feeling as strong as usual and you're immune system is more vulnerable to illness. Your metabolism fluctuates, resulting in chills, fatigue, emotional anxiety, stress, sleep disorders, and even dry skin. Yoga routines that balance vata focus on stabilizing the tissues, grounding the body, calming the mind, and enhancing strong bones and digestion.

THE EASY POSE

SUKHASANA

Sit on the floor (or on a cushion if this is more comfortable), legs outstretched and wide apart. Draw in your right heel and anchor it at your crotch. Draw in your left foot and tuck it under your right leg. Keep your spine erect. Extend both arms so your palms rest on your knees. Breathe in and then slowly exhale. Repeat for 5 to 10 breaths.

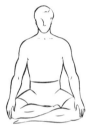

WIND-FREE POSE

PAVANMUKTA ASANA

Lie down on your back with your legs together and arms by your side, palms down. Bring your right knee to your chest, hugging it with both hands. Raise your chin toward your knee (or if that is too difficult, leave your head on the floor); keep your left leg relaxed. Breathe in and then slowly exhale. Hold for 5 to 10 breaths. Release and repeat on the other side. Then, contract your abdominal muscles to raise your legs about 6 inches off the floor. Raise both knees and hug them to your chest. Raise your chin toward your knees. If this is uncomfortable, keep your head on the floor. Breathe in and then slowly exhale. Hold the position for 5 to 10 breaths. Exhale completely and, holding the exhalation, contract your anus. Hold for a moment, then relax the anal region. Release your legs with an inhalation. Repeat the sequence 2 to 4 times.

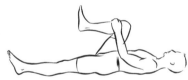

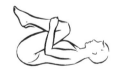

WARRIOR II POSE

VIRABHADRASANA

Stand straight with your hips square and your feet 3 to 4 feet apart. Breathe in, raising your arms straight out to your sides at shoulder level. Exhale and turn your right foot, knee, and leg to the right. Bend the right leg to 90 degrees, keeping your shin perpendicular to the floor and your hips facing squarely forward. Keep your right knee over your right heel. Keep your left leg and knee straight but not locked and turn you left foot slightly inward. Lengthen your lower back, opening your chest forwards and upwards. Breathe in and then slowly exhale. Repeat for 5 to 10 rounds of breathing. Then slowly release. Repeat the pose on the other side. Repeat the entire sequence 2 to 4 times.

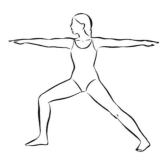

STOMACH LOCK

UDDIYANA BANDHA

Stand with your hips square and your feet 3 to 4 feet apart. Bend your knees and squat, placing your hands on your knees, fingertips facing in. Inhale, then exhale forcefully through an open mouth. Hold your breath, close your mouth, and tuck your chin into your chest. Suck your abdominal muscles back, up, and under your rib cage. Continue to hold the lock for 5 to 7 counts. Release your abdominal muscles. Inhaling, straighten your legs and come up to a stand. Exhaling, bend forward and hang loose. (Please note that holding the breath is contraindicated for heart issues.)

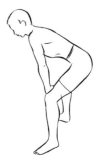

THUNDERBOLT POSE

VAJRASANA

Start by positioning yourself on your hands and knees, and then sit back on your heels and look forward. Keep your spine straight and place your palms on your thighs near your knee joints. Breathe in and then slowly exhale. Hold the position for 5 to 10 breaths, then exhale completely.

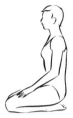

COBRA POSE

BHUJANGASANA

Lie face down. Position your legs together with the soles of your feet facing up and your forehead on the floor. Place your palms flat on the floor near your shoulders. Raise your head slowly, then the upper portion of your body to the pelvis (but keeping your pelvis on the floor). Arch your back as much as possible without placing pressure on your hands. Breathe in and then slowly exhale. Hold for 5 to 10 breaths, then release. Repeat 2 to 4 times.

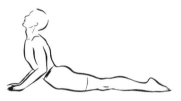

HALF LOCUST POSE

SHALABHASANA

Lie face down, arms by your side. Turn your chin toward but not touching the floor. Contracting the muscles of your waist and lower abdomen, raise both your legs off the floor as high as possible (or raise one leg at a time if that is too difficult). Breathe in and then slowly exhale. Hold for 5 to 10 breaths, then release. Repeat 2 to 4 times.

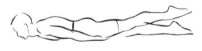

PLOUGH POSE

HALASANA

Lie flat on your back, legs together. Raise your legs slowly up and over your head until your toes touch the floor. Keep your knees straight but not locked and the palms of your hands flat on the floor, with arms outstretched. Take the hands toward the head and interlocking the fingers, place the palms behind

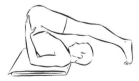

the scalp. Or if that is too difficult, use your hands to support your hips. Breathe in and then slowly exhale. Hold for 5 to 10 breaths, then release. Repeat 2 to 4 times.

CORPSE POSE

SHAVASANA

Lie flat on your back with your arms at your side, palms up, and your feet spread apart. Focus on your breath. Become aware of each part of your body and consciously relax it. Start with your right leg, working part by part from toes to groin, then relax your left leg in the same way. One at a time, relax your right and left hand and arm, working from fingers to shoulders. Then relax the front portion of your trunk, lower abdomen to upper abdomen, chest, and throat. Then relax your back, from lumbar region to mid back, neck, face, and the top of your head.

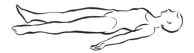

MEDITATIVE BREATHING

PRANAYAMA

This breathing exercise called *Suryabhedna* focuses on increasing heat in the body. Sit comfortably in a cross-legged position and slowly become aware of your breath. Take 10 natural breaths. Use your fingers to close your left nostril and inhale slowly through the right nostril. Retain your breath for as long as you comfortably can and then adjust your fingers to block the right nostril as you breathe out slowly through the left nostril. Build up breath-retention time with subsequent practice but only to a level of comfort, and never rush your out-breath. Ten to 15 minutes of this *pranayama* every day is extremely beneficial.

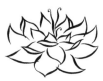

PITTA YOGA ROUTINE

Pitta imbalances are indicated by inflammation in the body and may manifest as excessive hunger or thirst and/or hypersensitivity, which may take the form of allergies, fevers, or indigestion. Negative and angry moods may also result. Yoga routines that balance pitta focus on creating coolness and on cleansing impurities in the blood.

STOMACH LOCK
UDDIYANA BANDHA

See page 86

BOW POSE
DHANURASANA

Lie face down, hands by your side, palms facing up, legs together. Turn your forehead to the floor, then, bending at the knees, raise your feet, bringing your heels as close to your buttocks as possible. Raise your head, keeping your chin on the floor, then reach back with your hands and grasp your ankles firmly. Pull your hands and legs together to raise your head, chest, knees, and thighs off the floor. Raise your clasped legs as high as possible, keeping the spine relaxed. Rest your entire body weight on your navel. Breathe in and slowly exhale. Hold for 5 to 10 breaths, then release. Repeat 2 to 4 times.

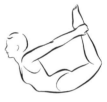

THUNDERBOLT POSE
VAJRASANA

See page 87.

FISH POSE

MATSYASANA

Sit on the floor with your spine straight, legs outstretched, feet together and toes pointed (or if this is too difficult, keep feet relaxed). Lean back and to the right, slightly shifting your position to place your right elbow on the floor behind you. Then, leaning slightly to the left, place your left elbow on the floor behind you. Slide your forearms towards your lower back (or sitbones), slowly lowering your head and back to the floor. Slide your hands under your buttocks, pressing your arms and elbows into the floor. Raise your torso and tilt your head back to arch your neck. Breathe in and slowly exhale. Hold for 5 to 10 breaths, then release. Repeat 2 to 4 times.

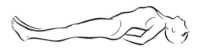

SPINAL TWIST POSE I

VAKRASANA

Sit on the floor with your legs together and outstretched, hands flat on the floor behind you. Bring your palms near your buttocks. Bend your right knee and place your right foot to the inside of your left knee. Twist your torso, bringing your left shoulder and hand towards your right knee, and tuck your right knee into your left armpit. Keep your right hand on the floor behind you. Twist your neck and body as far as is comfortable towards your right hand. Breathe in and then slowly exhale. Hold for 5 to 10 breaths, then slowly release. Repeat on the other side. Repeat the sequence 2 to 4 times.

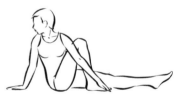

SPINAL TWIST POSE II

SULABHA MATSYENDRASANA

Sit on the floor, legs outstretched and ankles about 3 to 4 inches apart. Bend your right knee and bring it straight up to your chest. Bend your left knee, so that it points to the left, and keep it near the floor. Use your hands to position your left foot at or near your crotch. Move your right foot to the left side of your body, and use your left hand to place your right ankle behind your left knee. Hook your right big toe with your

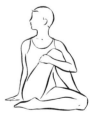

left index finger and tuck your right knee into your left armpit, or just place your left hand on your knee. Keep both buttocks on the floor. Twist your upper body to the right and put your right hand on the floor. If you can, bring your right hand around to your lower back. Breathe in and then slowly exhale. Hold for 5 to 10 breaths, then release. Repeat on other side. Repeat the sequence 2 to 4 times.

LEG-LIFT POSE

VIPARITAKARINI

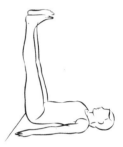

Lie flat on your back, legs together and outstretched and arms along your sides, palms down. Keeping your knees straight but not locked, contract your abdominal muscles to raise your legs about 6 inches off the floor. If this is too difficult, lie on your back with your buttocks against a wall and your legs raised above you, resting on the wall. Breathe in and then slowly exhale. Hold for 5 to 10 breaths, then release. Repeat the sequence 2 to 4 times.

PLOUGH POSE

HALASANA

See page 87

DOWNWARD-FACING DOG POSE

ADHO MUKHA SVANASANA

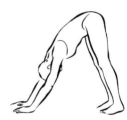

Lie face down, arms bent and palms flat on the floor at each side of your chest, fingers pointing towards your head. Tuck your toes under and lift up to your hands and knees. Exhaling, press your feet and hands into the floor and raise your buttocks, straightening your knees and pulling your thighs back. Do not lock your knees. Keep your spine straight. Extend your chest back towards your thighs. Keeping your elbows and knees straight but not locked, press your heels into the floor, push your hips up and pull your shoulders down. Breathe in and slowly exhale. Hold for 5 to 10 breaths, then release. Repeat the entire sequence 2 to 4 times.

CORPSE POSE

SHAVASANA

See page 88

MEDITATIVE BREATHING

PRANAYAMA

This breathing exercise, called *Shitali,* produces a cooling effect in the body. Sit comfortably in a cross-legged position and slowly become aware of your breath. Take 10 natural breaths. Partially protrude your tongue and then fold up the sides to form a long, narrow tube. Narrow the passage by further pressing the lips around the tongue. Inhale and receive the cold air passing through the tongue tube. Close your mouth and retain the breath for as long as you comfortably can. Exhale through both nostrils. Build up breath-retention time with subsequent practice but only to a level of comfort, and never rush your out-breath. Ten to 15 minutes of this *pranayama* every day is extremely beneficial for all *pitta* conditions.

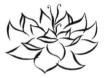

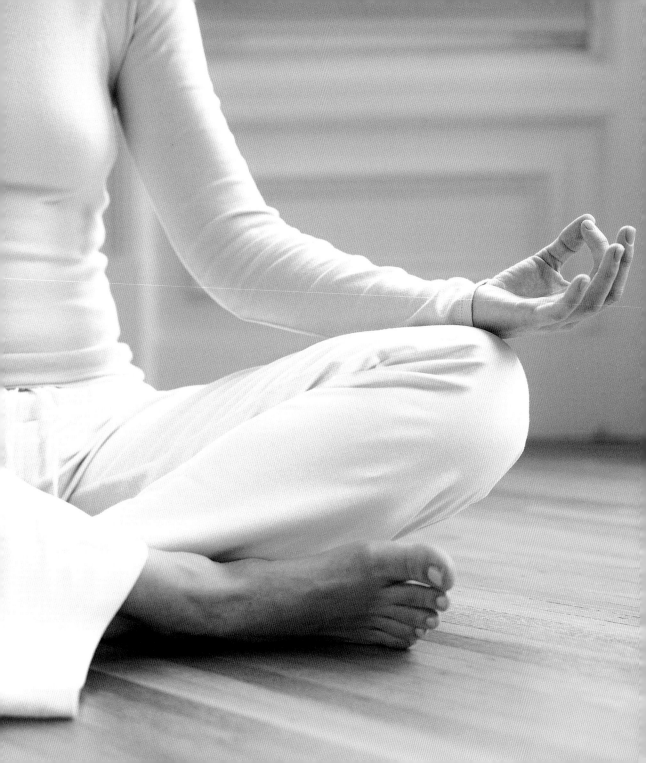

KAPHA YOGA ROUTINE

Kapha imbalances are generally indicated by swelling, congestion, and a general feeling of heaviness. Metabolism is slowed down, which leaves you feeling cold and sluggish all the time, and constantly perspiring. Yoga routines that balance kapha *focus on stimulating the mind and creating a feeling of lightness in the body.*

STOMACH LOCK
UDDIYANA BANDHA

See page 86

POSTERIOR STRETCH POSE
PASHCHIMOTTASANA

Sit on the floor, legs outstretched, arms alongside your body. Bending your trunk slowly, try to hook your fingers around your big toes (or grasp your calves or ankles if you are less flexible). Slowly bend farther forward, stretching your trunk along your thighs, and rest your face on your knees. Breathe in and then slowly exhale. Hold for 5 to 10 breaths, then release. Repeat 2 to 4 times.

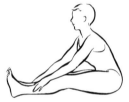

SEATED MOUNTAIN POSE
PARVATASANA

Sit on the floor, legs outstretched and spread as wide as is comfortable. Bend your right knee, and place your heel at your crotch. Bend your left leg and place your left foot under your right leg. Keep your spine straight. Flatten your palms together at your diaphragm, just below the middle of your chest and above your abdominals, projecting your elbows outwards. Raise your joined palms along the center line of your body to level of lips, then nose, then forehead, then above head, lengthening towards the sky. Your upper arms should touch your ears. Experience the pull from hips to fingertips. Breathe in and then slowly exhale. Hold for 5 to 10 breaths, then release. Repeat 2 to 4 times.

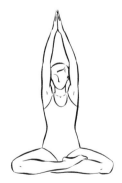

SPINAL TWIST POSE I

VAKRASANA

See page 90

CAT POSE

MAHARJASANA

Sit on your heels with your knees hip-width apart and toes on the floor. Position your palms on the floor in front of you at shoulder-width distance, and lean forward, bringing your hips up over your knees. Inhale, relax your trunk, and stretch your head and neck backwards, curving your spine and pressing towards the floor as far as is comfortable. Close your eyes and relax your stomach. Exhale, lower your head and neck, and raise back up, this time arching your spine as far as is comfortable. Release, relax your neck, and hang your head down, drawing your chin to your chest. Repeat 5 to 10 times.

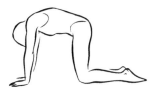

PALM TREE POSE

TAADASANA

Stand with your feet hip-width apart, hands at your sides. Raise your arms in front of you to shoulder height, palms facing down. Continue to raise your hands above your head while also raising your heels slowly. Stretch your arms fully, with your upper arms hugging your ears and your palms facing each other. Keep your heels together and balance. Breathe in and then slowly exhale. Hold for 5 to 10 breaths, then slowly release. Repeat 2 to 4 times.

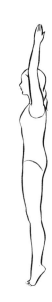

ADAPTED WHEEL POSE

PARIVARTACHAKRASANA

Stand with your feet hip width apart, hands at your side. Slowly raise both arms sideways to shoulder height. Bend towards your left side, still facing front. Drop your left arm to rest along your left thigh. Stretch your right arm above your shoulder, keeping it near your right ear, and slowly bend at the waist to your left, taking care not to strain yourself. With your right foot firmly on the floor, stretch upwards toward your right fingertips. Breathe in and then slowly exhale. Hold for 5 to 10 breaths, then slowly release. Repeat on the other side. Repeat the sequence 2 to 4 times.

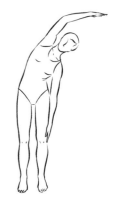

CAMEL POSE

USTRASANA

Kneel with the tops of your feet on the floor and your body straight and tall. Exhale and press your pelvis forward, leaning back gradually and lifting your chest. Reach back to your feet and grasp your heels, or just rest your hands on the back of your pelvis. Lean your head back, keeping your thighs perpendicular to the floor. Breathe in and then slowly exhale. Hold for 5 to 10 breaths, then slowly release. Repeat 2 to 4 times.

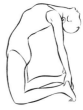

BOAT POSE

NAUKASANA/NAVASANA

Lie face down, chin to one side and hands at your side. Turn your forehead to the floor, bring your palms to chest level, and then stretch your arms ahead of you, palms down. Contracting the muscles of the buttocks, waist, back, and neck, raise your upper body from abdomen to fingertips while raising your lower body from abdomen to toes. Raise all parts high, keeping your elbows and knees straight but not locked. Breathe in and then slowly exhale. Hold for 5 to 10 breaths, then slowly release. Repeat 2 to 4 times.

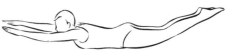

METABOLIC ASANA SERIES

This series of poses is designed to raise your heart rate and create the heat that *kaphas* need. Stand with your feet 3 to 4 feet apart, arms lifted to your sides at shoulder height and toes turned out. Bend your arms and point hands up to the sky. Exhale and squat, then inhale and straighten to stand. Keep your back straight and your abdomen tight. Repeat this 10 times. Jump your feet together and squat all the way down to the floor. Keeping your palms strong on the floor, exhale and jump your feet backwards, straightening your legs, raising your buttocks into downward-facing dog (page 91). Then inhale and jump your feet forward, returning to the squat position with your feet between your hands. Exhale and jump your feet back one more time into the downward-facing dog position. Jump your feet together or walk your hands back to your feet. Repeat the squat and downward-facing dog series 10 times. Straighten your legs and slowly stand upright. Repeat the entire sequence 3 to 7 times.

MEDITATIVE BREATHING

PRANAYAMA

This breathing exercise, called *Kapalbhati,* cleanses the nasal passages in the head and improves functioning of the diaphragm. Sit back on your heels, hands resting loosely on your knees, and slowly become aware of your breath. Take 10 natural breaths. Open your mouth very slightly. Expand your abdomen while inhaling and contract your abdomen while exhaling. Quickly alternate inhalation and exhalation, with accompanying expansion and contraction of the abdomen, to strongly activate your abdominal muscles for 30 breaths. This completes 1 round. Rest and repeat tor 30 breaths. Two to 5 rounds of this *pranayama* performed every day is extremely beneficial for addressing *kapha* imbalances.

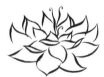

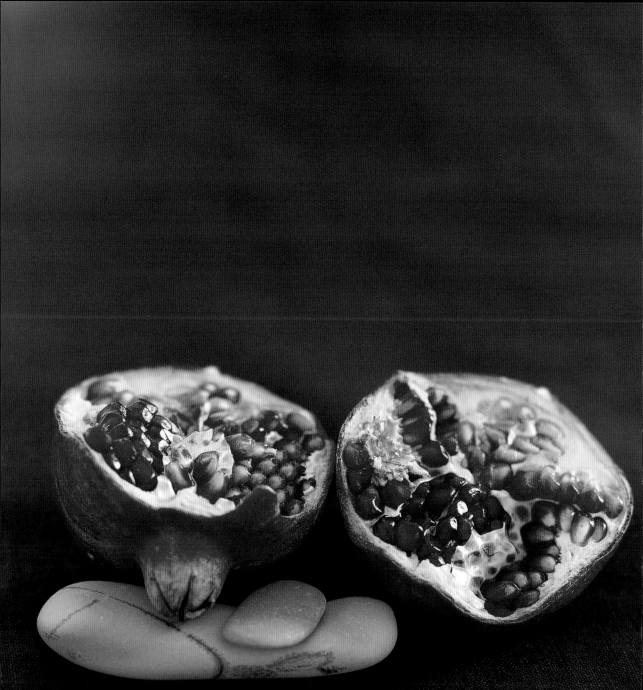

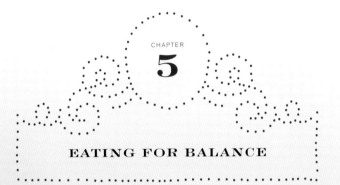

EATING FOR BALANCE

We all know that eating properly is crucial to good health. With the principles of Ayurveda, we can go even further in understanding how attention to diet can improve the quality of our lives. According to Ayurveda, everything about our eating habits has a strong effect on our mind and body—not only which foods and herbs we eat, but also the amount we eat, the timing of our meals and snacks, and the combinations of flavors all influence our well-being. The food we eat can have medicinal and therapeutic effects beyond mere sustenance. When we eat well, in every sense, we maximize our vitality *(ojas)*. Ayurveda recommends whole, nutritious foods and eating patterns that are tailored to balance your *dosha* type.

Poor digestion, stemming from an unbalanced diet, is one of the first signs of ill health. Indigestion disturbs *doshas* at their core, in the gastrointestinal tract. When our diet is off balance, not only are food nutrients not easily absorbed, but they can also accumulate as toxins. We all feel the effects of poor digestion differently: *kapha dosha* imbalances originate in the upper digestive tract (i.e., the stomach), *pitta* imbalances prey on the mid-digestive tract (i.e., the small intestines), and *vata* imbalances are felt in the lower digestive tract (i.e., the colon).

There is no "Ayurveda diet," and there are no "bad" foods in Ayurveda—there is only the idea of balance. A harmonious diet balances not only nutritional qualities, but also tastes and even the heating or cooling energetic effects a food has on us after it is digested. (Heating foods are those that are stimulating, such as black pepper, cooling foods are those that are sedating or can produce sluggishness, such as bread. *Sattwic* foods, such as almonds, create mental clarity and balance.) It takes into account individual items such as fruits, meats, and vegetables as well as the meals that they combine into once cooked. While there is an emphasis on fruits and vegetables, and many Indians are vegetarian, Ayurveda in itself does not prescribe vegetarianism. In fact, a whole array of meats and fish are emphasized in the ancient texts. But Ayurvedic doctors do recommend a pure and close to nature *(sattwic)* diet with plenty of fresh fruits, vegetables, nuts, and seeds combined with herbs and spices that will purify and balance the mind and body.

.:.:.:.:.:. **THE SIX TASTES (RASAS)** .:.:.:.:.:.

Understanding the concept of *rasa*, or taste, is critical for understanding the nutritional as well as the medicinal value of foods. In Ayurveda, there are six different tastes, each of which has a postdigestive effect on the *doshas* that influences the way we feel and how much energy we have. Most foods are a combination of more than one taste. In the West, we think of a balanced meal as one which combines fiber, carbohydrates, proteins, and fats, but in Ayurveda, a balanced meal is one that comprises all six tastes. We can tailor each meal to *dosha*-specific needs by having more of some tastes than others. We can then further customize the diet for corrective benefits. A healthy person is able to enjoy all of the six tastes, but if we have an imbalance, or *vikruti*, we sometimes develop an aversion to foods with similar qualities as the *doshas* that are imbalanced. These foods are then no longer palatable, no longer medicinal, and can even become bad for us. For example, if you have too much *pitta*, then spicy foods and chiles may not be appealing to you. To restore balance, a change of diet is always key. The positive and negative influences of each taste are detailed below.

SWEET

Foods with a sweet taste are calming and soothing to the system. Their grounding qualities balance *vata* and their cooling qualities balance *pitta*. But taken in excess, these foods will imbalance *kapha*, creating heaviness and slowing digestion. Sweet foods include not just sugar- and honey-based foods but also butter, milk, sesame seeds, fruits and vegetables with a naturally sweet taste (such as bananas or yams, and carbohydrates such as oats, rice, or wheat bread.

SALTY

Foods with a salty taste are warming and enhance digestion. Their warming qualities balance *vata* but taken in excess, they can disturb *kapha* and *pitta*, leading to water retention and inflammation. Salty foods include ketchup, dried or salted pickles, salted chips and other snack foods, and soy sauce.

SOUR

Foods with a sour taste stimulate digestion. Their warming qualities balance *vata* but taken in excess, they will disturb *kapha* and *pitta*, increasing body weight and skin sensitivity. Some examples are yogurt and buttermilk, pineapples, raw tomatoes, and fermented foods such as vinegar and pickles.

PUNGENT

Foods with a pungent taste decongest the body, increasing digestion. Their drying and heating properties balance *kapha*, but taken in excess, these foods can disturb *pitta* and *vata* by creating excess heat and dryness inside the body. Pungent foods include mustard, raw onions, and wasabi, and hot spices like chile peppers, caraway seeds, and black pepper.

BITTER

Foods with a bitter taste create lightness and clarity. They balance *kapha* and *pitta*, but taken in excess, they aggravate *vata*, inducing dryness in the skin. Examples of bitter foods are bitter melon, aloe vera, dark leafy green vegetables like spinach or mustard greens, and chicory.

ASTRINGENT

Foods with an astringent taste create lightness. Their cooling properties balance *pitta* and their drawing properties balance *kapha*, but taken in excess, these foods can disturb *vata*, leading to dryness and flatulence. Examples of astringent foods are pomegranates, cabbage, apples, and chickpeas.

For a meal to be balanced, it is important that we pay attention to the order in which we experience the six tastes. The six tastes digest in a specific order based on *doshas*. Sweet and salty tastes both are digested in the stomach, the first part of our gastrointestinal tract, by the *kapha dosha*. Therefore, these foods should be eaten first. Sour tastes are digested in the small intestine by the *pitta dosha*. These should be eaten next. Pungent, bitter, and astringent tastes are digested in the colon by the *vata dosha* and should be eaten last.

In the West, meals are typically served in courses. But in India small portions of food representing each of the six tastes are put together on large platters called *thalis*. That way, diners can pick and choose what food to eat in the preferred order and also adjust the intake of the tastes according to the *doshas* they are aiming to balance.

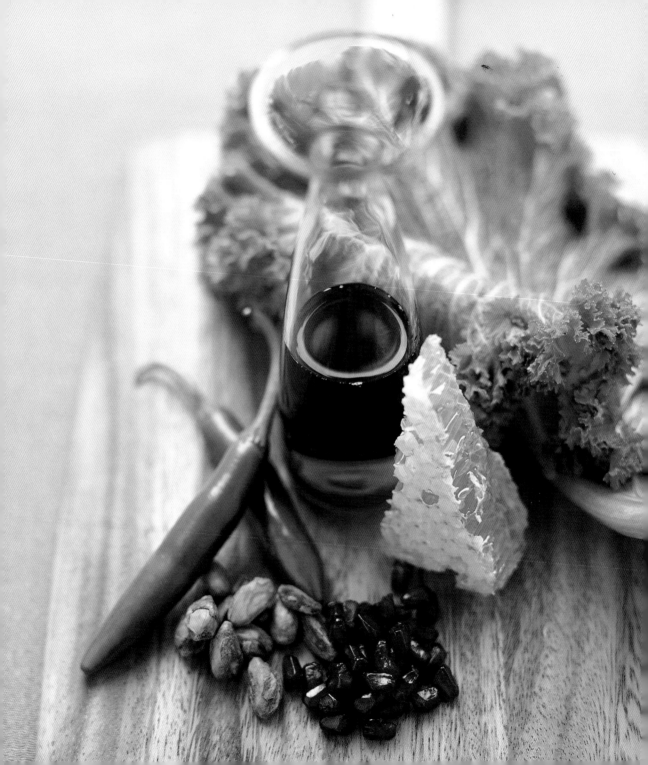

TIPS FOR PERFECT DIGESTION

Our constitution, or dosha, is affected by not just our food intake, but also by how we eat—how we feel when we eat and how long we take to have a meal, even when we snack. Follow the simple principles below to ensure optimal digestion.

1. Maintain a state of calm while eating. Eating under stressful circumstances turns your body into a pressure cooker, causing fermentation of the food in your digestive tract. This causes toxins to be absorbed into the bloodstream and even creates gas. Stress includes anything that takes away enjoyment from eating, from watching violent TV shows to discussing difficult situations.

2. Condition yourself to drinking water that is slightly warm or at room temperature, rather than ice cold water, as this dampens *agni,* or the "digestive fire" responsible for digesting food efficiently for maximum *ojas.* Avoid any water right before your meal; it is better to have water between meals. If possible, have two warm glasses of water upon rising and a glass of warm water or herbal tea following meals.

3. Chew your foods completely, without rushing. Foods that are not completely chewed and broken down in the mouth make for harder work for the stomach. This often leads to pain and discomfort during or right after your meal.

4. Make lunch the largest meal of the day. Digestive power is strongest when the sun shines directly overhead, so lunch should be your main meal, as foods have the best chance of being most efficiently digested. This is also the best meal to involve more complex foods. In the morning and evening, our system tends to be more sluggish. Therefore, breakfast and dinner should be smaller and be comprised of easily digestible foods, such as fruits for breakfast and lightly cooked vegetables, stews, and soups for dinner.

5. Eat nutritious, whole foods. Canned or overprocessed foods that have lost their color and flavor will have also lost their nutritional value. Also be careful how much you cook your fresh foods, especially vegetables. Indian chefs will tell you that when it comes to food, what you see is what you get—the more you can see the colors of different foods in your *thali,* the more nutritious your meal will be. Select foods that are whole and organic. These have more raw vitality, and can best balance your *doshas* in the way that nature intended them to.

6. Adjust food quantities according to your *dosha. Vata* types have a smaller food intake capacity but a more rapid metabolism. They often need four to five smaller meals in a day to give them the vital energy that keeps them functioning optimally. *Pitta* types have a strong metabolism and do well with three regular meals in a day. *Kapha* types have a slow metabolism, and should eat two to three meals in a day and avoid snacking.

7. Do not eat until after you have digested your previous meal. Eating too soon after your last meal causes bloating, acidity, and gas. While we all have different rates of digestion, rule of thumb tells us that we have completely digested a meal when we feel a sensation of lightness both physically and emotionally. This could be anywhere from two to four hours after a meal, but be sure to think about how you feel rather than look at the clock.

8. Eat sensible portions. It's easy to be lured by the appeal of gourmet foods and eat more than is appropriate. Starving ourselves for a trendy diet is just as bad. At each meal, the volume of our food should equal one *anjali,* or about two handfuls. This fills most of the stomach, the rest being left empty to allow food to mix freely with digestive juice and *vata* energy to push it down through the digestive tract. Fasting is not prescribed in Ayurveda—it weakens *ojas* energy, compromising strength and complexion.

9. Follow your meal with digestives. India has a wonderful tradition of digestive munchies, called *mukhwas,* eaten at the end of a meal to help encourage digestion. Eating 1 teaspoon of *mukhwas* is a great after-meal ritual. Make your own from equal parts of sesame seeds, whole cumin seeds, and fennel seeds, and keep the mix in a jar in a cool, dry place.

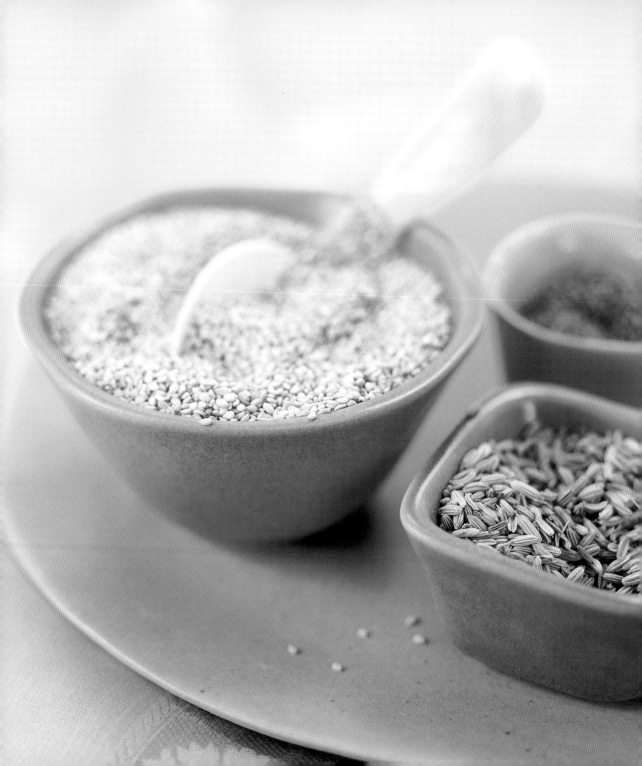

Once you've identified your *dosha*, experiment with making a few changes to your diet that will help keep your body in balance. Of course, you won't be able to stick to these guidelines all the time, but being conscious of your body's natural tendencies is a great way to help control your moods, keep your energy up, and maximize your *ojas*.

VATA

Eat many small meals throughout the day to help sustain your energy level.

Eat warm, cooked, light foods with sweet, salty, and sour tastes. Avoid cold foods like ice cream and chilled purees.

Moisten dry or raw foods, breads, and omelets with ghee (see page 77), oil, or butter.

Avoid caffeine in excess.

Substitute brown sugar, honey, or maple syrup for white sugar.

Avoid gassy, bloating foods such as beans and soda. If you really enjoy beans, cook them with ghee and digestion-aiding herbs such as ginger, cardamom, cinnamon, cilantro, and dill.

Favor root vegetables and leafy greens for your vegetable consumption. Do not eat them raw, however; cook them, preferably with ghee or sesame oil.

Eat plenty of fleshy fruits such as peach, mango, and papaya. Drink plenty of citrus, fruit, and vegetable juices.

Do not mix different types of animal proteins such as fish and eggs, milk and meat, or turkey and shellfish.

Avoid low-fat diets. *Vata* types need the nutritious quality of fats.

Sip a specially blended *vata* tea (available at specialty stores) to help regularize digestion in the colon, or try salty lassi (an Indian beverage made from yogurt and water).

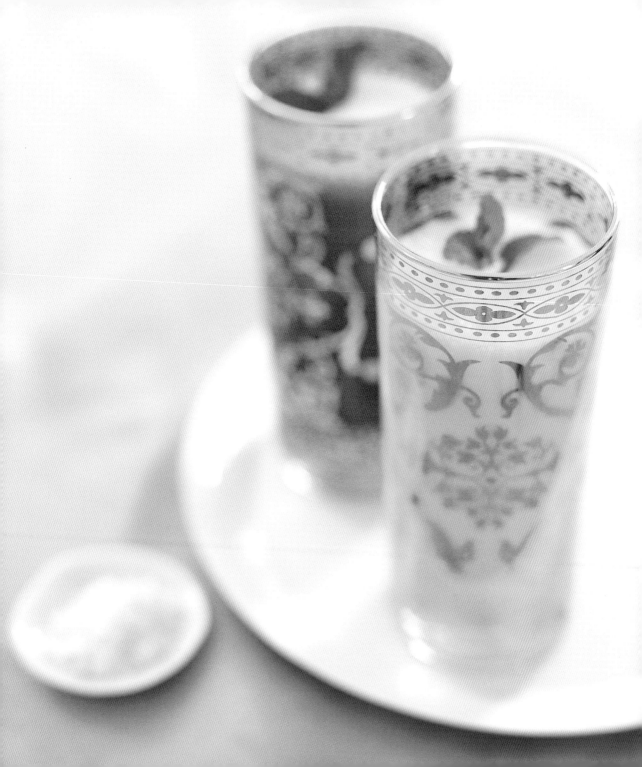

PITTA   Eat three meals a day with lunch as your main meal.

Eat cooling and light foods with sweet and bitter tastes.

Avoid caffeine, alcohol, salt, or spices in excess.

Substitute brown sugar for honey, maple syrup, or white sugar.

Avoid yeasted grains, such as breads. Choose flatbreads and rice, spread with ghee (see page 77) and sprinkled with cooling digestive herbs such as cilantro, parsley, and dill.

Favor leafy greens for your vegetable consumption. Bitter greens are your best bet and quite plentiful through the year. Vary your selection, choosing from spinach, mustard, kale, and collard greens.

Eat plenty of sweet fruits such as sweet cherries, red grapes, or figs. Avoid sour citrus fruits and juices, such as grapefruit. Drink plenty of green drinks such as parsley, celery, or wheatgrass juice. An excellent drink for *pittas* is equal parts vegetable juice and coconut milk, enhanced with 1 teaspoon of either aloe vera or spirulina.

Avoid foods such as mustard, hard yellow cheeses, red meats, tomatoes, and eggplant. These heating foods will further incense the fiery *pitta* qualities.

Sip a specially blended *pitta* tea (available in specialty stores) to balance acidity and soothe your stomach, or drink milk or cranberry juice.

KAPHA   Make sure that dinner is the lightest meal of the day and try to eat no later than sunset. Soups and light vegetable stews make ideal dinners.

Eat warm, dry, light foods with bitter, pungent, and astringent tastes.

Avoid heavy oils and butters or fried, fatty foods. Opt for lighter oils such as olive or canola oil.

Avoid caffeine and sugar in excess.

Avoid heavy, congestive foods that are difficult to digest such as pastas, breads, and cakes.

Eat plenty of dark leafy green and brightly colored vegetables like celery, carrots, spinach, and tomatoes.

Eat plenty of citrus fruits and berries. Drink citrus, fruit, and vegetable juices.

Avoid more than three meals in a day and maintain a gap of at least four hours between meals. Also, avoid snacking between meals.

Avoid high-protein diets for extended periods.

Sip a specially blended *kapha* tea (available in specialty stores) to balance digestion in the stomach and prevent discomfort during and after meal-times. Also try salty lassi (an Indian beverage made from yogurt and water), buttermilk, or lemonade.

Flush your system with water throughout the day.

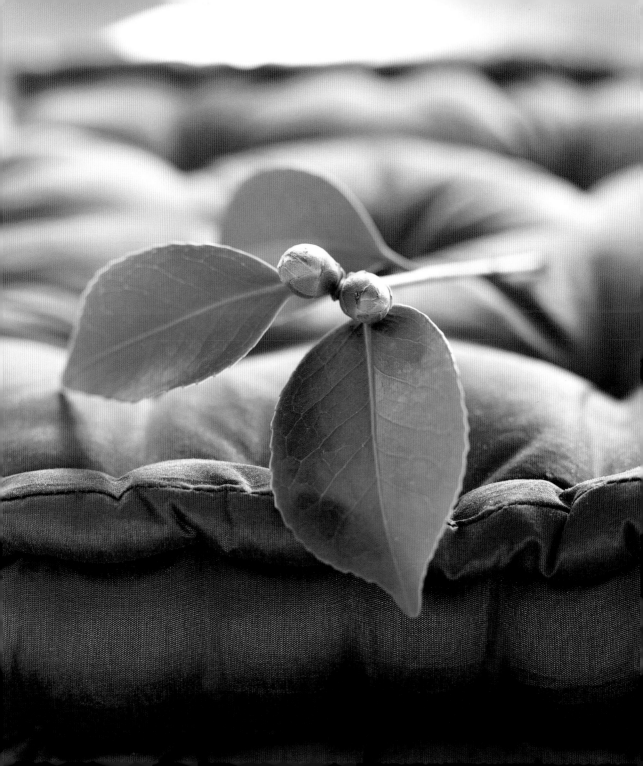

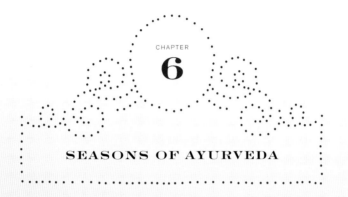

SEASONS OF AYURVEDA

While we practice our Ayurvedic *dinacharya*, or daily self-care regimen,
year-round, it is important that we try to match our lifestyle rhythms to
those of the season and the geography around us. Just like a person, the
environment and seasons are characterized by the three *doshas*, each of
which is more active and influential at different times of year.

    The change in Ayurvedic seasons affects the balance of our *doshas*.
While any one *dosha* might dominate our constitution, remember that we
are each made of all three, and that these might be thrown off balance by
the strong influence of the *dosha* of the season. If we don't shift our nutritional and lifestyle patterns to balance what is happening in the environment, the *dosha* within us that is the same as the *dosha* of the season will be
thrown off course. This doesn't mean that we have to completely reinvent
our life several times a year, but merely that we should make small changes
to live in harmony with the seasons. While the supermarket can provide all
foods all year round, it is wise to eat warming foods in winter or cooling
fruits in the summertime. Try eating fresh produce, fruits, and vegetables
that are available through farms and suppliers close to where you live to be
sure that you are in tune with the season. You might also want to change

your yoga routine—the secret here lies in our ability to adjust and adapt accordingly the needs of the seasons' *dosha*. Also, since each of the *doshas* has a tendency to become aggravated during the season prior to that of its peak influence, it is ideal to undergo a cleansing program to bring this *dosha* back into balance at the onset of its season of influence. Ayurveda suggests three such detox retreats or cleansing programs during the year— at the onset of the season where each *dosha* is at peak influence.

The Ayurvedic year can be roughly divided into three seasons (which overlap with the traditional four seasons of the Western calendar), each of which has its own influencing *dosha*. The *vata* season runs from Western fall into winter, when the weather turns cold and dry. At this time of the year we can eat heavier, warming foods with plenty of natural oils and protein. Avoid salads and drying foods, such as chickpeas or dry lentils during this season, as these will exacerbate *vata*. Winter meals prepared with nourishing foods such as nuts, meats, and warm and creamy soups, stews, or casseroles are ideal for the *vata* season. Exercising indoors is preferable at this time of the year to avoid the onslaught of wind and cold temperatures which can further exacerbate *vata*. We all tend to feel more tired at this time of the year, so slow down and make things easy on your-self. It's ideal to conduct a *vata* detox retreat (see facing page) in October or November, right at the onset of *vata* season.

The *kapha* season runs from late winter to spring. Flowers begin to bud during this cool, damp time of the year. Eat light, fresh foods such as vegetable soups and light stews during this season. Avoid dairy, ice cream, and excess oils as they will naturally aggravate *kapha*. In many cultures, this is the time of the year for spring festivals, which wake people into action after the sleepy wintertime. It's a good idea to lead an all-around more active lifestyle now, whether that means taking brisk walks or keep-ing yourself mentally and physically occupied with reading or aerobic activity; avoid napping. This is the season for undertaking projects. *Kapha* detox retreats conducted in late January or February, before the onset of *kapha* season, will help you combat congestion, allergies, and sluggishness during this time of the year.

The *pitta* season runs from summer into early fall. This is the time when the sun is strongest overhead and the fire element is at peak influence. To compensate, eat colder, sweeter foods and cool drinks. Avoid hot, spicy foods and excess alcohol, as these will create inflammation. Choose moderate exercise that tones the muscles without causing you to overheat, such as walking and swimming. During these months, avoid inverted postures, such as headstands, in your yoga practice. And remember, the days are long now, so get plenty of rest and, if possible, take short naps. This will help you stay calm and collected in many situations. As with the other seasons, it is ideal to undergo a *pitta* detox retreat in June or July, before you are into the thick of the season.

.:.:.:.:. SEASONAL DETOX RETREAT .:.:.:.:.

A detoxification program is ideal for eliminating *dosha* imbalances that naturally build through the seasons. Classical Ayurvedic detoxification is called *Panchakarma*, and it is an intensive program of invasive therapies that require the supervision of a physician. While *Panchakarma* is beneficial, it is not easily available, nor essential for maintaining strong *ojas*, unless your *doshas* are quite severely out of balance and causing illness. Checking into an Ayurvedic spa to undergo a short detox program based on *Purvakarma*, the nutritional and body therapies that support *Panchakarma*, three times a year is ideal, as the staff will be able to guide you with treatments, food, yoga, and other activities that will help restore balance and maximum vitality. However, given the time and expense, it's good to know how to follow your own simple detox program at home. The program described below is designed as a simple, three-day program that can be easily done at home over a weekend. The key to a successful detox is to stay focused and shut out the rest of the world, allowing you both emotional and physical release. The detox guidelines below are ideal for any *dosha* season, or can be customized with foods and herbs for the season at hand. Remember to use your judgment—detoxing is not advised for children, pregnant or nursing mothers, or people who have been diagnosed with an illness or are taking strong medication.

THE WEEK BEFORE

To prepare for your detox, it is important to loosen and liquefy toxins and bring them to the superficial tissue layers. For seven days before your retreat, follow your normal personal-care routine, but start every day by drinking a $1/4$ to $1/2$ cup of warmed ghee (see page 77). Follow this with an astringent liquid like orange juice or hot water with fresh lemon juice to help take away the aftertaste (this will also help encourage bowel elimination.) Try to get into the habit of emptying your bowels soon after consuming this drink. In addition, drink 8 to 10 cups of warm water through the day.

FRIDAY

Begin the detox retreat with a cleansing ritual. Start your day with ghee and hot lemon water per the previous seven days. Then, using a tongue scraper or just a toothbrush, scrape your tongue from back to front 6 to 7 times, followed by your normal personal-care routine. Eat as lightly as possible through the day; try to avoid heavy proteins, carbohydrates, sweets, and fried foods. Also avoid sodas, coffee, and tea. As with the previous seven days, drink 8 to 10 cups of warm water through the day.

EVENING MEAL

When you come home from work, eat a light meal, such as a seasonal vegetable salad and a bowl of vegetable soup. On the side, have some toasted rye bread without butter. Drink a cup of triphala tea following your meal: boil 1 teaspoon of triphala herbs (see page 40) in 4 ounces of hot water. This gentle laxative will help remove toxins throughout the digestive system. Be sure not to sweeten the tea. Eat dinner by 6 PM, so that you will

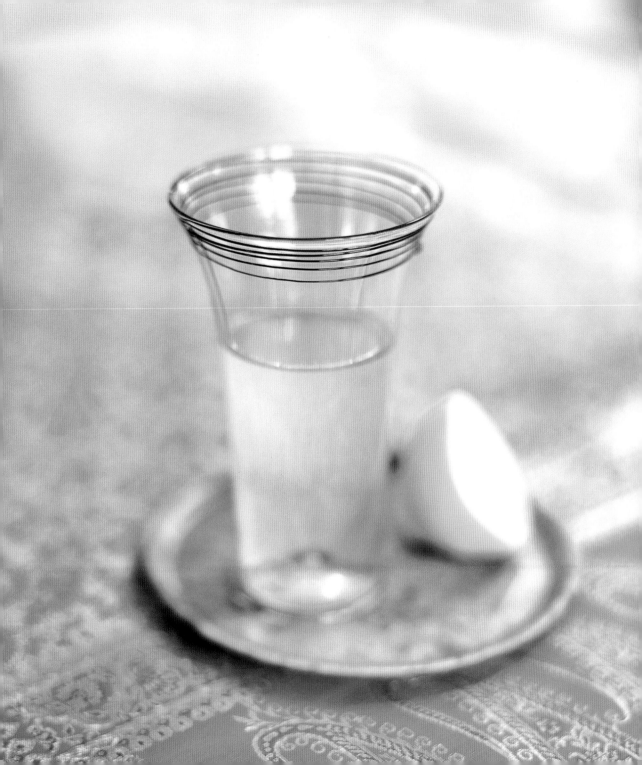

have plenty of time to sip herbal tea through the remainder of the evening. Note: *vatas* should replace the salad with a fistful of cooked seasonal vegetables dressed with plenty of sesame oil and fresh herbs and seasonings. *Vatas* may spread ghee (see page 77) on the rye toast. *Pittas* should make sure that their vegetable soup has an even mixture of green and colored seasonal vegetables.

FACE AND NECK MASSAGE

Giving yourself a twenty-minute face and neck massage with a *dosha* facial oil will help to ease headaches and relieve tension and anxiety (see page 52). Throughout the massage, focus on releasing tension in your neck by letting go of your head and allowing it to become heavier and heavier, creating pressure against your hands.

MEDITATIVE BREATHING (PRANAYAMA)

In a well-ventilated room, sit comfortably in a cross-legged position on the floor or in a straight-backed chair. Close your eyes and relax your body. Try to shut out distractions from your mind so that you can completely focus on the breath. If your mind wanders, observe the thought, let it pass, and then bring your attention back to your breath. As you become aware of your breath, breathe in for a count of three, hold briefly, and then breathe out for a count of six. If you are able, then increase the length of your in-breath and out-breath, but make sure that you always maintain the 1:2 proportion with a brief hold between each complete round. Continue several rounds this way—at least fifty rounds or five minutes, whichever comes first. Next, breathe normally for another five minutes or so, focusing on your breath without counting. Finally, focus on the part of your nose where the coolness of your in-breath meets the warmth of your out-breath. Remain focused on this and then think of a positive emotion. Nurture it and resolve to further it. Remain focused on this emotion for a few minutes before you gradually come out of your meditation.

Avoid television or loud music today. Try to avoid reading, as it is important that you focus inward and clear yourself of thoughts and stimuli. Go to sleep early, as you will need to wake up early tomorrow. Prepare a copper vessel with an infusion of herbs in warm water and leave to stand overnight (see pages 130-131 for herbs).

SATURDAY AND SUNDAY

Throughout these two days, drink water and herbal teas; aim to drink 10 to 12 glasses of water and as much herbal tea as you would like. Be sure to drink warm, not iced, water; iced water dampens the digestive fire *(agni)* that is responsible for efficient digestion.

WAKING UP

On both these days, wake up slowly, joyously remembering that the day is dedicated to you. Make yourself a hot lemon drink by squeezing the juice of half a lemon into 1 cup of herb-infused water from the copper vessel you prepared the night before. Heat the water and sip it slowly to begin your body's natural detox processes. Go to the bathroom and try to empty your bowels, but remember not to strain or push yourself.

NASAL CLEANSING AND TONGUE SCRAPING

Splash your face and eyes with cold water. Then, using a *neti* pot (see page 83), cleanse both nostrils with 1 tablespoon of mustard oil mixed into 1 potful of *dosha* herbal tea and a pinch of salt (see page 83 for complete instructions). Use at least two potfuls per nostril. Using a tongue scraper or toothbrush, scrape your tongue from back to front at 6 to 7 times to get rid of toxins.

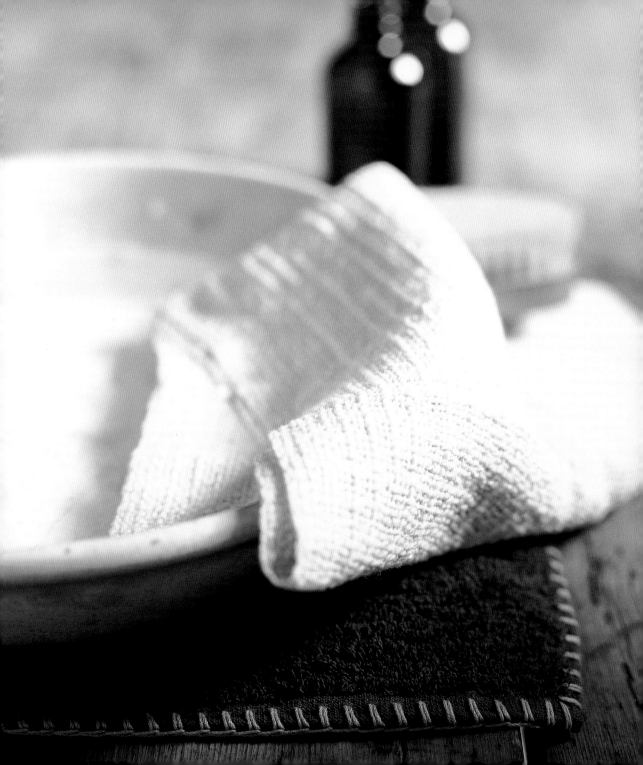

Give yourself an invigorating dry skin-brushing with a rough towel or natural loofah, to help slough off the dead skin cells that can clog your pores, helping your skin to breathe better. Skin-brushing stimulates the lymphatic system and helps to revitalize the skin. Brush all over, starting with your arms and legs and working inward towards the heart. Applying only as much pressure as is comfortable, brush until your skin becomes warm, but do not overdo it and cause your skin to redden excessively; five minutes or so is plenty. Follow the brushing with an *abhyanga* massage (see page 47) and feel the oils penetrate into the pores. *Pitta* types might be a little more sensitive, and everyone should be careful not to brush on broken or irritated skin.

MORNING YOGA

Start off Saturday and Sunday with a rejuvenating yoga practice. Follow the appropriate yoga routine for the *dosha* of the season, as outlined in Chapter Four. End with alternate nostril breathing, a yogic technique that harmonizes your energy and strengthens respiration.

In this *pranayama*, the out-breath is twice as long as the in-breath and so efficiently clears waste products from the lungs and body. Don't strain your breath, but focus on keeping it long, steady, and deep, building rhythm and intensity as you go along.

Close your right nostril with your right thumb and exhale completely through your left nostril. Inhale through your left nostril to a count of four. Close your left nostril with your ring finger and little finger, holding your index and middle fingers to the bridge of your nose. Hold for a count of four. (If you can, build this up to a count of eight.) Release your right nostril, exhaling completely for a count of eight. Close the right nostril and keep both nostrils closed for a count of four (or eight if you can). Repeat the sequence on the other side. This sequence is 1 round. Repeat the breathing technique for at least 15 rounds, or better still, for 10 to 15 minutes.

For the first meal on each of these two days, eat a large bowl of fruit salad with a tall glass of freshly squeezed orange juice or *dosha* herbal tea. This meal will help the liver begin ridding the body of accumulated waste matter. *Vata* types benefit from adding a handful of sesame, sunflower, or pumpkin seeds for constitutional warmth. *Pitta* types might find orange juice too acidic, and may substitute *pitta* tea or any other fresh fruit juice of the season. You may also prepare a blended fruit smoothie in place of the salad: in a blender, combine a large banana with $1/2$ cup of your choice of seasonal fresh fruits and $1/2$ cup of water to thin it out.

DETOX SPA TREATMENTS

If you are visiting a spa for Ayurvedic detoxing, take advantage of available face and body treatments while you are there, as they help loosen and expel toxins. If you are detoxing at home, undertaking these treatments will aid the rejuvenation experience. Follow the suggestions below for a comprehensive Ayurvedic home-spa experience.

SATURDAY

Face and Body Scrub with *Ubtan:* Prepare a cleansing *ubtan* scrub (see pages 54–56). Work the scrub all over your face and body to improve circulation and tone slack muscles. Rinse with warm water.

Herbal Steam: This is a great practice to eliminate toxins. Steam your face over a bowl of hot water combined with two handfuls of seasonal herbs (see pages 130–131) for about 10 minutes. Hold your face at least 12 inches above the water and tent your head and the bowl with a towel to prevent the steam from escaping. (*Vata* types, who may find steam alone too drying, can apply a little sesame oil to the face and neck before steaming.) Pat your face dry and splash with tepid water to refresh the skin. Run a hot shower to generate steam and rest in the steam 7–10 minutes to purify the skin of the body as well.

Lepa mask: This mask absorbs impurities from the skin. Mix together a mask (see pages 66–68) and apply it all over the face and body. Leave the mask on for about 15 minutes and try to remain as still as possible (*Vata* types may add a few tablespoons of sesame oil to the mixture if they find it too drying). Rinse with warm water.

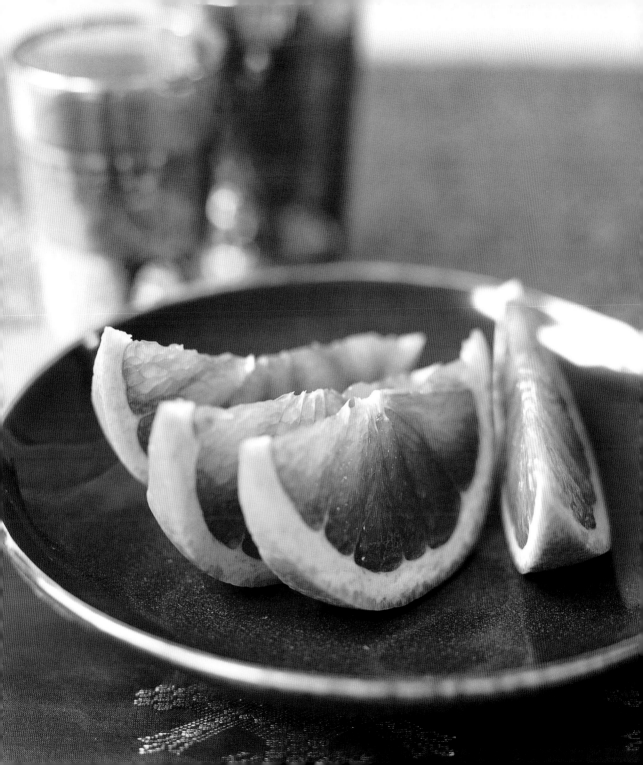

Rinse: Rinse your face and body with a mixture of 1 tablespoon cider vinegar diluted in 4 ounces of water. The cider vinegar is an excellent natural toner.

Moisturize: Massage your face and body with aloe vera gel for *pittas* or heavy whipping cream for *vatas* and *kaphas* to soften and refresh your skin.

SUNDAY

On Saturday, you cared for your skin; on Sunday, focus on hair, hands, and feet.

Hair and Scalp: Cleanse and oil the hair (see pages 73–74). This will help condition, detoxify, and supply nutrients to your hair and scalp. Leave the oils in for as long as possible. Rinse thoroughly, then apply a nourishing protein mask to your scalp made from 1/2 cup yogurt, 1 tablespoon lemon juice, 1 egg, and 2 tablespoons brahmi powder (if available; see page 40). Leave this mask on for about 20 minutes, then rinse thoroughly.

Hands and Feet: With a loofah or rough hand towel, gently massage your hands and feet to increase circulation. Then soak your hands and feet in a tub of warm water infused with any of your favorite essential oils. Use a pumice stone to ease out any rough areas on the feet. Warm 3–4 tablespoons of ghee (see pages 77) and rub generously into your hands and feet, massaging per the instructions outlined in Chapter Three. This will moisturize, relieve tension, and prevent water retention. If you have cold extremities, keep your hands and feet warm for a resting period by wrapping them in a hot wet towel that has been wrung dry and wrapped in another dry towel.

DOWN TIME

During your detox program, spend part of the morning as you like—reading an interesting book, listening to music, writing in your journal, gardening, painting…the choices are endless. It is important though to spend time unwinding and doing what you want to rather than what you think you should do.

LUNCH

After your morning yoga and spa therapies, enjoy a large raw salad made with fresh vegetables of the season (*vata* types should have a cooked vegetable salad). Choose from the *dosha* balancing herbs and spices listed in Chapter Five and the Ayurvedic Pantry (see page 39) to add flavor. Eat your lunch slowly and mindfully, focusing on the flavors and textures of the ingredients. While you eat, reflect on the view from your window, or even the sight of indoor plants and flowers, to unlock the mind.

REST

Rest is important to calm the mind and allow the physical body to deal with fatigue as it detoxes. After lunch take some quiet time to listen to music, read, or take a short nap for half an hour to an hour if you are sleepy. If you are tired but cannot fall asleep, then simply rest your mind and body by lying down and emptying your mind of thoughts.

EXERCISE

Your detox retreat will be enhanced by a brisk walk, preferably in the open air so that you can breathe natural oxygen directly into your lungs (during the chill of *vata* season, or in northern climates, you may use a treadmill). Staying aware of good posture, warm up by starting out at a slow pace and then build to a brisk pace. Keep your chest out, swing your arms wide, and breathe through your mouth. Walk for 20 to 30 minutes, with the goal being 1 hour. If you prefer other types of exercise, consult the chart on pages 130–131 for modes of exercise appropriate for the *dosha* of the relevant season.

MUSICAL MEDITATION

When you begin to feel the effects of your detox, musical meditation is ideal. Put on some of your favorite music. Try to choose music that evokes the positive emotions for the *dosha* of the season (see pages 130–131). To do this, select music that reminds you of the emotion you are focusing on. For example, during a *vata* seasonal detox program, choose music that is calming and provides focus. During a *pitta* seasonal detox program, choose music that reinforces love and respect for the people you know. Music can be of any genre—jazz, classical, popular, world music, different instrumental types—but avoid loud, jarring, disturbing sounds or controversial music of any kind. Spend at least half an hour listening to the music and thinking about a time or situation in your life when you most felt this emotion. This could be when you were young, or it could be recently. Try to take yourself deeper into this emotion and plan how you can carry it through to new experiences in your life. Feel your state of mind uplifted with this new positive emotion.

DIGESTIVE MEDITATION AND CARE

This is an ideal time to tune into your digestive system and become familiar with it. Place your hands first on your stomach and become aware of any internal movements, feelings, or sounds. Do the same with your small intestines in your midriff area and then with the area under your navel, or colon. Mentally prepare for your next meal by noticing whether you are hungry or not. Resolve to eat only as much as you need to fill three-quarters of your stomach (this typically translates to about as much food as will fit into both your cupped hands). Using a little bit of oil, massage your stomach in round circles, moving clockwise. This will help ease digestion of the last meal and prepare for the next.

DINNER

Dinner during detox should consist of steamed vegetables. Use fresh, green seasonal vegetables, the greener the better. For extra flavor, add fresh herbs such as rosemary, basil, parsley, and sage, or pine nuts, sesame seeds, or pumpkins seeds. *Vata* types may add a bit of oil to their vegetables. As with lunch, eat slowly and mindfully, allowing complete digestion. An hour or so after dinner, follow with triphala tea (see page 40).

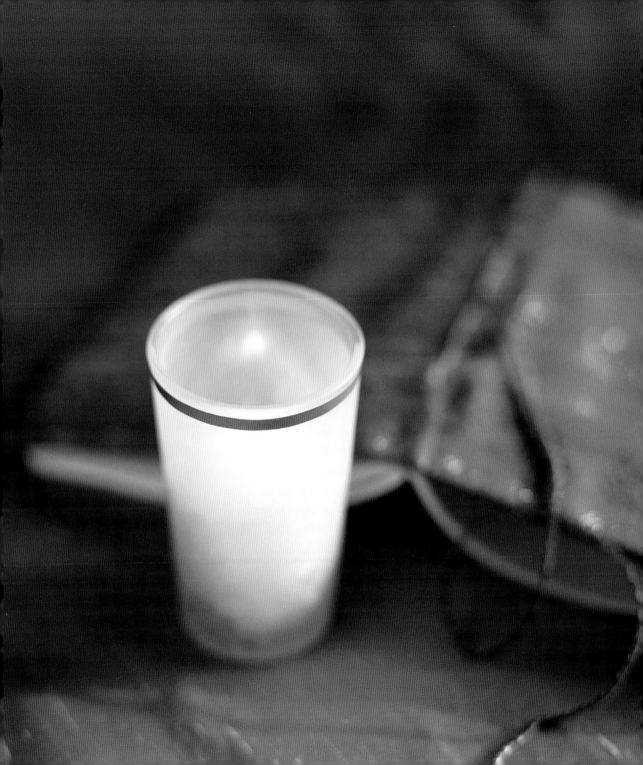

AMUSEMENTS

This is your time to spend doing things that are creative and mindful, yet relaxing. These can be anything from light reading to working the Sunday crossword to needlepoint or organizing photographs. Do something that you enjoy and perhaps do not often get a chance to do during your regular weekly schedule. Think about why you enjoy the activity and the kind of satisfaction or creative stimulus you derive from it. Be thankful for this time to pursue it.

BATH AND BEDTIME

Run a bath prepared with ingredients to balance the *dosha* of the season (see pages 59–60). In the *vata* season, it is better to have a warm shower rather than a bath. If you like, add candles, fresh flowers, and music to aid relaxation. As you soak in the bath, close your eyes and breathe deeply, releasing tension with each exhalation. Keep yourself warm after the bath and go to bed, relaxed and at peace.

AFTER THE WEEKEND

As you come out of your detox program, don't return immediately to your regular eating habits. Eat light foods such as vegetable soup, kichadi (a mixture of rice and lentils cooked together with digestive herbs and ghee), or a light rice and mung beans dish. Avoid heavy foods like meat, dairy, and bread for at least a day or two, as they will be hard to digest right after your detox retreat.

Coming out of the detox retreat, you will more than likely feel tired, perhaps a little heavy-headed and somewhat "out of it." Your moods and emotions may be heightened, so you might feel extra weepy, chatty, quiet, or low. It is important to recognize these as signs of active detoxing and not worry about them as unusual or associated with feeling ill. As with diet, it is important then that we gradually readjust to normal life and not rush back into a frenzied pace of existence.

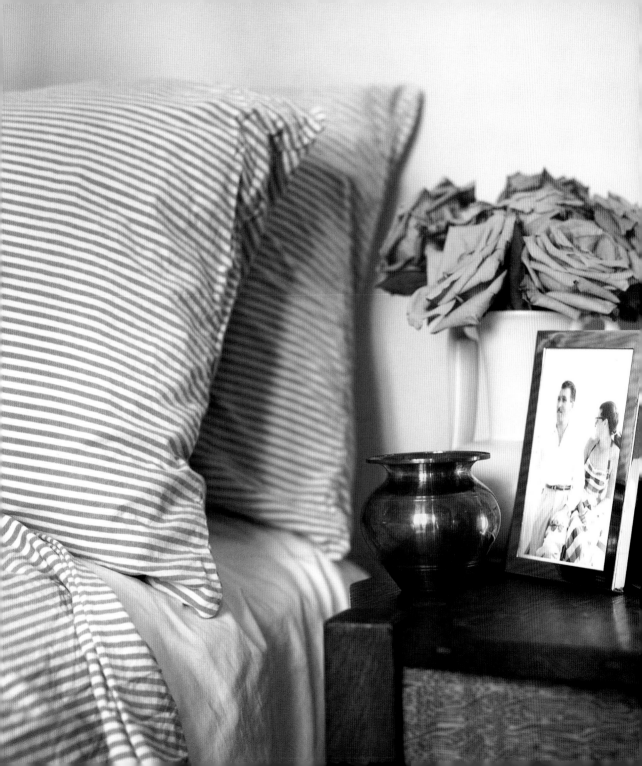

DOSHA SEASONAL DETOX GUIDELINES

Each season's detox calls for particular elements, whether specific thoughts to meditate on or specific herbs to use for cleansing and massage. This chart will help you determine which dosha *dominates the season you are experiencing and the appropriate remedies to balance your* prakruti *in that season. For more information about facial, massage, and body therapies, see Chapter Seven.*

VATA SEASON (FALL TO LATE WINTER)

MODES OF EXERCISE	Tai chi, dance
POSITIVE EMOTIONS FOR MEDITATION	Focus, calm
HERBAL TEAS	*Vata* tea, ginger tea
FACIAL AND BODY ABHYANGA*(MASSAGE) OIL*	*Vata* oils
HERB-INFUSED WATER FOR COPPER VESSEL	Ginger and fennel
FACIAL, MASSAGE, AND BODY THERAPIES	Day 1: *Abhyanga, mukhralepa*
	Day 2: *Tanlepa, taila seka, Shiro dhara*
AROMATHERAPY OILS	Sandalwood, oilbaum, jatamansi
HERBS FOR FACIAL STEAMING	Ginger and mixed herbs
MOISTURIZERS	Heavy whipping cream

PITTA SEASON (SUMMER TO EARLY FALL)

MODES OF EXERCISE	Swimming, skiing, basketball
POSITIVE EMOTIONS FOR MEDITATION	Love, respect for others
HERBAL TEAS	*Pitta* tea, peppermint tea
FACIAL AND BODY ABHYANGA*(MASSAGE) OIL*	*Pitta* oils
HERB-INFUSED WATER FOR COPPER VESSEL	Coriander
FACIAL, MASSAGE, AND BODY THERAPIES	Day 1: *Abhyanga, Shiro dhara*
	Day 2: *Tanlepa, Shiro abhyanga, mukhralepa*
AROMATHERAPY OILS	Sandalwood, rose, neem, jasmine
HERBS FOR FACIAL STEAMING	Coriander and basil
MOISTURIZERS	Aloe vera gel

KAPHA SEASON (LATER WINTER TO SPRING)

MODES OF EXERCISE	Aerobics, cycling, rowing
POSITIVE EMOTIONS FOR MEDITATION	Organization, creative stimulation
HERBAL TEAS	*Kapha* tea, ginger and lemon tea
FACIAL AND BODY ABHYANGA*(MASSAGE) OIL*	*Kapha* oils
HERB-INFUSED WATER FOR COPPER VESSEL	Ginger and turmeric
FACIAL, MASSAGE, AND BODY THERAPIES	Day 1: *Abhyanga, mukhralepa*
	Day 2: *Udvartana, Shiro abhyanga*
AROMATHERAPY OILS	Cedarwood, juniper, neem
HERBS FOR FACIAL STEAMING	Fennel and parsley
MOISTURIZERS	Yogurt

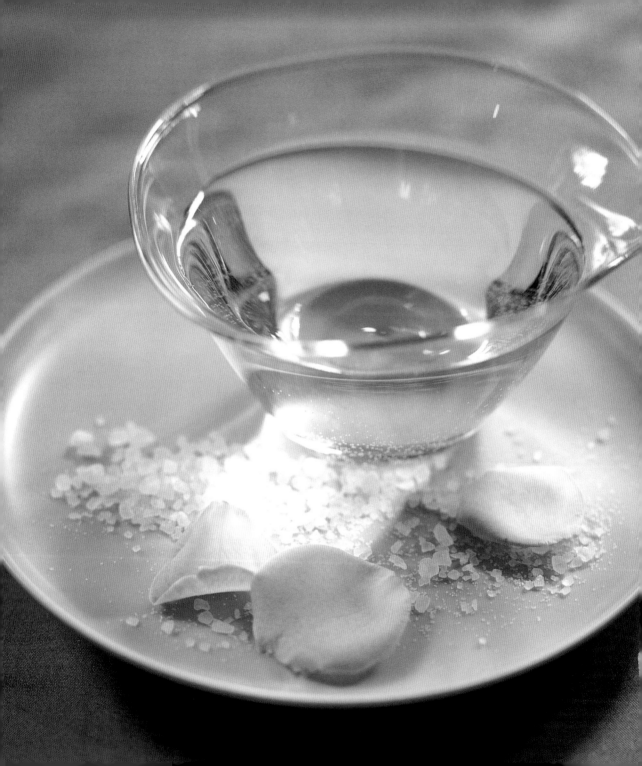

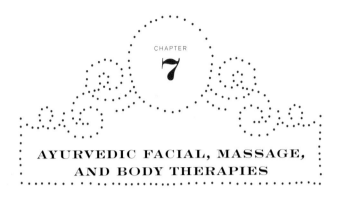

CHAPTER

7

AYURVEDIC FACIAL, MASSAGE, AND BODY THERAPIES

Ayurveda tells us that both the physical body and the emotional body can be rejuvenated through massages, facials, and body therapies. Some of these treatments call for year-round practice, and others work as seasonal pick-me-ups. While this book is intended as a means to comfortably and easily embrace Ayurvedic practices on your own, a trip to an Ayurvedic spa or wellness center, with expert technicians, can provide an excellent education. If you don't live near an Ayurvedic spa, try seeking one out for a yearly or seasonal getaway. While the treatments described in these pages are ideally performed as maintenance on a regular basis, a single session at a spa can also be quite effective. Ask the practitioner to focus on your *dosha*-balancing needs, or the *dosha*-balancing needs of the season, and don't be afraid to ask questions.

.:.:.:.:.:. **MASSAGE WITH THERAPEUTIC OILS (ABHYANGA)** .:.:.:.:.:.

Abhyanga literally translates as "oil application." Ayurveda provides various oil massage therapies that relax and detox the mind and body. While self-*abhyanga* benefits us every day, *abhyanga* received from a seasoned Ayurvedic technician with appropriate herbal oils prepared from medicinal plants truly meets your body's unique needs. Various styles of *abhyanga* are available, each distinguished by their own regional Indian flavor. Sometimes the technician will stimulate *marma*, the vital energy points that awaken immune responses. Often, more than one technician will massage your body, rhythmically moving with silent communication like a traditional Indian dancer.

.:.:.:.:.:. DHARA (OIL THERAPY) .:.:.:.:.:.

Dhara means "flow"—in this case, the flow of therapeutic oils. Of all dhara therapies, *Shiro dhara* is the most well known for its ability to relieve emotional and physical tension. Warm, herbal-infused streaming oil is poured onto the third eye (the area between the eyebrows) and over the forehead to relinquish the negative energies that bring on depression, nervousness, sadness, and fatigue. Other *dhara* therapies include *Chakra dhara*, a treatment that flows herbal oils onto the body's subtle energy centers such as the navel, solar plexus, and throat to link our physical, mental, and emotional interactions. In *Pizichil*, or *Taila seka*, *Rasayan* oil, a rejuvenating herbal oil, is simultaneously flowed onto and massaged into the body to rejuvenate the nervous system and relieve inflammation in the joints.

.:.:.:.:.:. UDVARTANA (CLEANSING) .:.:.:.:.:.

Udvartana eliminates toxins created by smoking, water retention, and environmental poisons. This vigorous massage with fragrant herbal powders stimulates the lymphatics and cleanses the blood, the skin, and the tissues that lie beneath it. Typically, *udvartana* is combined with an *abhyanga* that helps dislodge impurities and an herbal steam bath that encourages the body to release them.

.:.:.:.:.:. **TANLEPA (HERBAL PLASTER)** .:.:.:.:.:.

Lepa translates as "medicinal plaster." *Lepa* therapy helps reduce inflam-
matory swellings and draws out impurities from inside the body to the skin
surface. *Tanlepa* combines three different Ayurvedic therapies. First, a
dosha specific oil massage is provided along the *nadis*, or energy channel.
Then warm oil is poured rhythmically up and down the body's energy
meridians. The body is then covered with *dosha*-specific herbs and
wrapped in a foil blanket to maintain warmth as the body releases heat.

.:.:.:.:.:. **SHIRO ABHYANGA (SCALP AND SPINE MASSAGE)** .:.:.:.:.:.

Another critical component of Ayurvedic therapies, this therapy for the
central nervous system provides a deep massage of the head, neck, and
back starting from the base of the spine to release toxic energy upward and
out of the crown chakra (energy release point). A completely indulgent experience, it heals through the central chakras and *marmas* (vital energy
points), and helps correct the posture. With this physical adjustment, we
receive amazing mental clarity and awareness.

.:.:.:.:.:. **MUKHRALEPA (DOSHA FACIAL)** .:.:.:.:.:.

Ayurvedic skin-care therapies focus on cleansing and purifying from
within, by balancing your *dosha* from its origin in the digestive system.
Mukhralepa is a holistic facial treatment that combines five ancient
Ayurvedic beauty techniques traditionally used by brides for their wedding
day, all for the purpose of cleansing, detoxifying, and nourishing the system to enhance beauty from within. Perfect for maintaining skin tone or
targeting areas of aging or acne, this treatment includes *Shiro dhara*
(herbal oil flow on the third eye), facial *marma abhyanga*, and the use of
herbal applications, and foods that result in glowing, radiant skin, and
emotional balance.

AYURVEDIC TERMS

Ama – Bodily toxins, or undigested food matter.

Asana – Yoga posture.

Ayurveda – The "science of life," India's ancient system of wellness.

Brahma – Creator of the universe, one of the three main gods in the Vedic tradition. He is believed to have spoken in the *Rig Veda* (see facing page).

Chakras – Energy centers of the body. The seven major chakras are the top of the head, the forehead, the throat, the heart, the solar plexus, the navel and lower abdomen, and the base of the spine.

Dinacharya – Daily routine.

Diwali – The annual Hindu Festival of Lights that marks the new year. The goddess Lakshmi is celebrated during this festival.

Dosha – An energetic force that is a combination of two of the five elements of nature, and part of the makeup of each person. The three doshas are *vata* (earth and air), *pitta* (fire and water), and *kapha* (water and earth).

Ganges River – The holy river that runs through the northern Indian plains.

Jalneti – Nasal cleansing practice (see page 83).

Lakshmi – Goddess of wealth. She is the consort of Lord Vishnu, and epitomizes the capacity of the *kapha dosha:* grounding, stability, and prosperity.

Lord Krishna – Hindu god, an incarnation of Lord Vishnu who expounded the famous *Bhagvad Gita (The Divine Song).*

Marma – Vital points on the physical body where life energies are believed to be concentrated.

Ojas – The vitality, or essence, of the mind and body.

Panchakarma – Classical Ayurvedic clinical detox regimen, involving a complex of procedures that requires clinical supervision.

Parvati – Vedic goddess of strength. She is the wife of Lord Shiva, and epitomizes the capacity of the *pitta dosha:* strength and power.

Prakruti – Natural state of balance; mind-body constitution.

Prana – The breath, life force.

Pranayama – Yogic breathing practice.

Purvakarma – Ayurvedic massage, nutritional, and body therapies that loosen toxins in the body so that they can be eliminated naturally.

Radha – A shepherdess who was a devotee of Lord Krishna.

Rajas – The mental attributes of kingliness.

Rasayan – Rejuvenatives that build and strengthen bones and tissues, and prevent aging. Ashwagandha, shatavari, brahmi, and ghee are all examples of *Rasayans*.

Rig Veda – The oldest of the four books of spiritual knowledge of India. Ayurveda was discussed in these books before being organized into its own system of health care.

Ritucharya – Seasonal routine.

Sanskrit – The language of ancient India and the ancient writings on Ayurveda.

Saraswati – Vedic goddess of knowledge, consort of Lord Brahma. She is the goddess who epitomizes the capacity of the *vata dosha*—learning, creativity, and art.

Sattwa – The mental attribute of purity, balance.

Shiva – The destroyer of negativity, one of the three main gods in the Vedic tradition.

Svedana – Heat therapy. One of the most common forms is the use of steam heat.

Tamas – The mental attribute of dullness, inertia; toxic-minded.

Ubtan – A purifying legume-and-herb cleansing paste that is applied to the skin to purify the blood and circulatory system.

Vikruti – Fluctuation or imbalance of physical and emotional elements which disrupts a person's natural well-being.

Vishnu – The preserver of the universe, one of the three main gods in the Vedic tradition.

Yoga – A holistic Vedic science related to Ayurveda that improves health and vitality by harmonizing the mind, breath, and body. Ayurvedic texts describe the components of yoga as ethical practices, rules or punctuality of daily routine, postures or physical exercises, breathing routines, sensory practices, and meditation. Postures and breathing are most predominantly practiced as yoga today.

REFERENCES

Ashtanga Hridayam of Vagbhata. Translated by a Board of Scholars. Delhi, India: Sri Satguru Publications, a division of Indian Books Center, 1999.

Kulkarni, P. H. *Ayurveda Soundaryam.* Delhi, India: Sri Satguru Publications, a division of Indian Books Center, 1998.

Nimbalkar, Sadashiv P. *Yoga for Health and Peace.* Bombay, India: Yoga Vidya Niketan, 1992.

Raichur, Pratima and Marian Cohn. *Absolute Beauty.* New York: HarperPerennial, 1997.

Rastogi, R. P. and B. N. Mehrotra. *Compendium of Indian Medicinal Plants.* 5 vols. New Delhi, India: National Institute of Science Communication, 1960–89.

Sharma, Dr. Ram Karan and Vaidya Bhagwan Dash. *Carak Samhita.* 6th ed. Varanasi: Chowkhmbha Sanskrit Series Office, 2000.

RESOURCES

INDEX

ACKNOWLEDGMENTS

This book has been a labor of love. Hopefully it will be as inspiring
to read as it was to write. My thanks go to:

Feroza Unvala, for her unique ability to visualize my thoughts; Anjali Joshi, our yoga guru, for supporting my interest in pursuing the study of yoga, Ayurveda, and the Vedic sciences; Kathryn Keller, my colleague at the Institute of Health and Healing in San Francisco, who consulted on the yoga section of this book.

My agent Felicia Eth, who encouraged me to take all the steps to bring this project to fruition; my editor Lisa Campbell, for deciding to take a chance on this book; Sara Schneider, France Ruffenach, and Sara Slavin for making it as beautiful as it could be.

My friends and coworkers at Ayoma, who work to support the cause of Ayurvedic education and self-care in the West, and remind me every day of the ambassadorial goals we are collectively working towards.

Gopal Krishan Vij, my late grandfather, who first taught me about inner beauty, and encouraged me to write down everything I wanted to say to the world; Neeraj Hora, who encourages me to look for the beauty in situations that might not outwardly appear beautiful; Veena and Rajinder Malhotra, who have always believed in me; Ilya Devi and Arya Vir Hora, who inspire me to maximize *ojas* every day; Sushma Hora who interested me in the healing properties of medicinal plants.

All teachers, practitioners, and missionaries of Ayurveda. It is your dedication that inspires people to seek out this life-changing philosophy in the first place.

All the folk interested in Ayurveda. I hope that you may share this wellness philosophy with others.